Lecture Notes in Statistics 86

Edited by S. Fienberg, J. Gani, K. Krickeberg, I. Olkin, and N. Wermuth

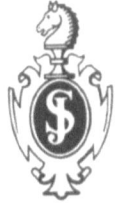

Werner Vach

Logistic Regression with Missing Values in the Covariates

Springer-Verlag
New York Berlin Heidelberg London Paris
Tokyo Hong Kong Barcelona Budapest

Werner Vach
Institut für Medizinische Biometrie
Abteilung Medizinische Biometrie und Statistik
Klinikum der Albert-Ludwigs-Universität
Stefan Meier Strasse 26
D-7800 Frieburg
GERMANY

Library of Congress Cataloging-in-Publication Data
Vach, Werner.
    Logistic regression with missing values in the covariates / Werner
Vach.
        p.   cm. -- (Lecture notes in statistics ; 86)
    Extended version of the author's thesis (doctoral) -- University of
Dortmund
    Includes bibliographical references and index.

    (Berlin : acid-free) : DM58.00
    1. Regression analysis. 2. Estimation theory. 3. Missing
observations (Statistics) I. Title. II. Series: Lecture notes in
statistics : v. 86.
QA278.2.V25 1994
519.5'36 -- dc20   94-247

Printed on acid-free paper.

© 1994 Springer-Verlag New York, Inc.

Softcover reprint of the hardcover 1st edition 1994

Camera ready copy provided by the author.

9 8 7 6 5 4 3 2 1

ISBN-13: 978-0-387-94263-6   e-ISBN-13: 978-1-4612-2650-5

DOI: 10.1007/978-1-4612-2650-5

Editorial Policy
for the publication of monographs

In what follows all references to monographs are applicable also to multiauthorship volumes such as seminar notes.

§ 1. Lecture Notes aim to report new developments - quickly, informally, and at a high level. Monograph manuscripts should be reasonably self-contained and rounded off. Thus they may, and often will, present not only results of the author but also related work by other people. Furthermore, the manuscripts should provide sufficient motivation, examples, and applications. This clearly distinguishes Lecture Notes manuscripts from journal articles which normally are very concise. Articles intended for a journal but too long to be accepted by most journals, usually do not have this "lecture notes" character. For similar reasons it is unusual for Ph.D. theses to be accepted for the Lecture Notes series.

§ 2. Manuscripts or plans for Lecture Notes volumes should be submitted (preferably in duplicate) either to one of the series editors or to Springer-Verlag, New York. These proposals are then refereed. A final decision concerning publication can only be made on the basis of the complete manuscript, but a preliminary decision can often be based on partial information: a fairly detailed outline describing the planned contents of each chapter, and an indication of the estimated length, a bibliography, and one or two sample chapters - or a first draft of the manuscript. The editors will try to make the preliminary decision as definite as they can on the basis of the available information.

§ 3. Final manuscripts should be in English. They should contain at least 100 pages of scientific text and should include
- a table of contents;
- an informative introduction, perhaps with some historical remarks: it should be accessible to a reader not particularly familiar with the topic treated;
- a subject index: as a rule this is genuinely helpful for the reader.

Dedicated to my teachers
Paul O. Degens and Günter Rothe

Acknowledgements

I would like to express my sincere gratitude to several people who have contributed to the rise and progress of this book. My colleagues at the Institute of Medical Biometry in Freiburg have always stimulated my work by presenting new examples of missing values in their daily work and by their comments on my proposals. My thesis advisor Martin Schumacher spent a lot of time on reading and discussing my drafts and he made a lot of valuable suggestions. Maria Blettner from the German Cancer Research Center gave me a deep insight into the problem of missing values in the analysis of epidemiological studies, provided me with several data sets, and was always interested in discussing new approaches theoretically and in examing their applicability in practice. My discussions with Margaret Pepe at the Hutchinson Cancer Research Center in Seattle were very fruitful and she pointed out a lot of open questions to me. The final revision of the manuscript was done during a stay at the MRC Biostatistics Unit in Cambridge and several discussions with David Clayton had some impact on Chapter 11. Walter Schill from the BIPS read a preliminary version carefully and gave several constructive comments. For the kind permission to use his data I am indebted to Hans Storm. Ina El-Kadhi contributed by typesetting major parts of the manuscript. Finally Magdalena Thöne supported my work by her absence and presence and by her valuable suggestions with respect to language and style. Many thanks to all of them and to those which I have forgotten to mention.

The support of this research project by the *Deutsche Forschungsgemeinschaft* is gratefully acknowledged.

Notice

This book is an extended version of the author's Ph.D. thesis accepted by the Department of Statistics, University of Dortmund.

Contents

1. Introduction

In many scientific areas a basic task is to assess the simultaneous influence of several factors on a quantity of interest. Regression models provide therefore a powerful framework, and estimation of the effects in such models is a well-established field of statistics. In general this estimation is based on measurements of the factors (covariates) and the quantity of interests (outcome variable) for a set of units. However, in practice often not all covariates can be measured for all units, i.e., some of the units show a missing value in one or several covariates. The reasons can be very different and depend mainly on the type of the measurement procedure for a single covariate and the type of the data collection procedure. Some examples should illustrate this:

- If the covariate values are collected by a questionnaire or interview, non-response is a typical source for missing values. It may be due to a true lack of knowledge, if for example a person is asked for certain diseases during its childhood, or to an intentional refusal. The latter is especially to be expected for embarrassing questions like alcohol consumption, drug abuse, sexual activities, or income.
- In retrospective studies covariate values are often collected on the basis of documents like hospital records. Incompleteness of the documents causes missing values.
- In clinical trials biochemical parameters are often used as covariates. The measurement of these parameters often requires a certain amount of blood, urine or tissue, which may not be available.
- In prospective clinical trials the recruitment of patients can last several years. Meanwhile scientific progress may discover new influential factors, which may cause the decision to add the measurement of the covariate to the data collection procedure. For patients recruited before this decision the value of this covariate is missing.
- If the measurement of a covariate is very expensive, one may restrict the measurement to a subset of all units.
- Even in a well planned and conducted study small accidents can happen. A test tube may break, a case report form may be lost on the mail, an examination may be forgotten, the inaccuracy of an instrument may be detected too late, etc. Each accident may cause a missing value.

The traditional theory for estimation in regression models gives no hint to deal with missing values in the covariates. The standard approach of most statistical software packages is Complete Case Analysis, i.e., all units with at least one missing value are excluded from the analysis. As the excluded units have a measurement of the outcome variable and some covariates, they still carry some information on the effect of these covariates. Hence Complete Case Analysis is wasteful of information. Especially small missing rates in several covariates can sum up to a substantial loss of data.

To overcome this inefficiency, one approach is to impute a guess for each missing value in order to achieve a complete data set. Several strategies to construct such guesses have been suggested. However, estimates of the variance of the estimated regression parameters from the artificially completed data set are invalid in general, because we have to correct for the variation due to guessing the imputed values. One approach is to assess this variance by repeated guesses; this is the basic idea of multiple imputation methods.

The emphasis of this book is on methods related to the classical maximum likelihood (ML) principle. It is well known from the basic work of Rubin (1976) that this principle can be applied in the presence of missing values, too. However, the handling of missing values in the covariates by the ML principle requires to specify the distribution of the covariates at least in part. Since a reasonable specification seems to be out of reach for most applications, semiparametric approaches avoiding this specification are of great interest. First suggestions have been recently made (Pepe & Fleming 1991, Carroll & Wand 1991, Reilly & Pepe 1993), but need to be investigated further.

In the first part of this book we examine three (semi-) parametric approaches for the specific situation of logistic regression with two categorical covariates and missing values in one covariate. In contrast to these sophisticated approaches, where theoretical results establish consistency of the estimates, we also consider some widespread approaches often resulting in asymptotically biased estimates. These approaches are Complete Case Analysis, imputation of estimated probabilities, regarding missing values as an additional category and omission of the covariate affected by missing values. The choice of logistic regression with two categorical covariates and missing values in one covariate is motivated by the following arguments:

- The logistic model is one of the most important tools in the analysis of clinical and epidemiological studies. Furthermore the relation between the regression coefficients and adjusted odds ratios allows a simple assessment of the bias of some methods of dealing with missing values.
- Contrary to continuous covariates categorical covariates allow to consider maximum likelihood estimation. Hence we can use maximum likelihood estimation in our comparison as the golden standard.
- Two covariates with missing values in one covariate is the most parsimonious model where we can expect the existence of methods superior to Complete Case Analysis.

In Chapter 2 we start with a summary of some basic properties of the logistic model and the estimation of the regression parameters in the complete data case. Chapter 3 is devoted to the discussion of missing value mechanisms. The essential point is the *missing at random* assumption, which excludes a dependency between the true covariate value of a potentially unobserved covariate and its observability. In Chapter 4 we describe several methods to deal with missing values; the presentation includes the discussion of basic statistical properties, the computation of the estimates and the estimation of asymptotic variance. For those methods yielding biased estimates of the regression parameters a first qualitative assessment of the bias is given. The comparison of the consistent estimation methods by means of asymptotic relative efficiency and the comparison of the asymptotic bias of the other methods is the topic of Chapter 5. Evaluations of finite sample size properties by means of simulation studies are presented in Chapter 6. The examples in Chapter 7 are selected in order to demonstrate some basic properties of the methods and differences between the methods. Because the *missing at random* assumption is essential for those methods superior to a Complete Case Analysis, we present in Chapter 8 a suggestion for a procedure examining the sensitivity of a single estimate against violations of this assumption.

In the second part of this book we consider generalizations of the approaches described in the first part. Chapter 9 starts with general regression models specified by a parametric family for the conditional distributions of the outcome variable. We restrict to the case of two covariates where only one is affected by missing values, but allow arbitrary scales of the covariates. Although it is rather simple to generalize the basic ideas, a theory establishing consistency and asymptotic normality and allowing the estimation of asymptotic variances is available only for special cases, for which references are given. A special section is devoted to the Cox proportional hazards model. Of highest practical interest is the generalization to situations with more than two covariates with arbitrary patterns of missing values. The basic difficulties of this step are described in Chapter 10. Chapter 11 is devoted to the special type of missing values due to a planned subsampling. We describe the relation of approaches used in this field and the approaches considered in this book. Chapter 12 presents two examples involving regression models with more than two covariates.

The problem considered in this book should be clearly distinguished from other related problems. First we consider only the situation, where the value of a covariate is *completely* unknown. We do not consider the case of censored, grouped or mismeasured covariate values, although some of the methods considered have a direct analogue for these problems (cf. Heitjan 1989, Carroll et al. 1984, Whittemore & Grosser 1986, Schafer 1987 and Carroll 1992). Second we only consider missing values in the covariates, not in the outcome variable. The latter problem is total different and exhaustively treated in the literature (e.g. Yates 1933, Bartlett 1937, Jarrett 1978, Dodge 1985).

A systematic investigation of methods to handle missing values in the covariates of a logistic regression model has not yet been provided in the literature. Some recommendations based on personal experience are given by Chow (1979); Yuen Fung & Wrobel (1989) and Blackhurst & Schluchter (1989) present some results from simulation studies.

Part I: Logistic Regression With Two Categorical Covariates

2. The Complete Data Case

The Model

Let be Y a binary outcome variable, X_1 a covariate with categories $1, \ldots, J$ and X_2 a covariate with categories $1, \ldots, K$. In a logistic model we assume

$$P(Y = 1 | X_1 = j, X_2 = k) = \Lambda(\beta_0 + \beta_{1j} + \beta_{2k}) =: \mu_{jk}(\beta) \tag{2.1}$$

with parameter restrictions $\beta_{11} = 0$ and $\beta_{21} = 0$. $\Lambda(x) := 1/(1 + e^{-x})$ denotes the logistic function. We consider the covariates as random variables, and parametrize their joint distribution by

$$
\begin{aligned}
P(X_1 = j) &=: \tau_j \qquad \text{and} \\
P(X_2 = k | X_1 = j) &:= \pi_{k|j} \; .
\end{aligned}
\tag{2.2}
$$

We collect the regression parameters to a vector $\beta = (\beta_0, \beta_{12}, \ldots, \beta_{1J}, \beta_{22}, \ldots, \beta_{2K})$ and the parameters describing the joint distribution of the covariates to $\tau = (\tau_j)_{j=2,\ldots,J}$ and $\pi = (\pi_{k|j})_{k=2,\ldots,K, j=1,\ldots,J}$. The cell probabilities

$$p_{ijk}^* := P(Y = i, X_1 = j, X_2 = k)^{1\dagger)} \quad \text{with } i = 0, 1; j = 1, \ldots, J; k = 1, \ldots, K$$

can now be expressed as

$$p_{ijk}^* = \mu_{jk}(\beta)^i (1 - \mu_{jk}(\beta))^{1-i} \pi_{k|j} \tau_j \; .$$

The logistic model (2.1) can also be expressed as assumptions about odds ratios to be constant within strata. With

$$\phi_{jk}^* := \frac{p_{1jk}^* p_{01k}^*}{p_{0jk}^* p_{11k}^*}$$

denoting the odds ratio between the j-th category of X_1 and the first category (which is the arbitrary chosen reference category) given $X_2 = k$, the assumption (2.1) is equivalent to

$$\phi_{jk}^* \equiv: \phi_j^*$$

and then $\phi_j^* = \exp(\beta_{1j})$ holds. Analogously with

$$\psi_{jk}^* := \frac{p_{1jk}^* p_{0j1}^*}{p_{0jk}^* p_{1j1}^*}$$

$^{1\dagger)}$ Symbols with an asterisk always refer to quantities defined in the complete data case

denoting the odds ratio between the k-th category of X_2 and the first category given $X_1 = k$, the assumption (2.1) is equivalent to

$$\psi_{jk}^* \equiv: \psi_k^*$$

and then $\psi_k^* = \exp(\beta_{2k})$ holds.

In the following we assume that we have n units with independent observations $(Y_r, X_{1r}, X_{2r})_{r=1,\ldots,n}$ distributed according to (2.2) and (2.1). These observations can be summarized in a $2 \times J \times K$ contingency table with entries

$$n_{ijk}^* = \#\{r \mid Y_r = i, X_{1r} = j, X_{2r} = k\} .$$

Maximum Likelihood Estimation

The contribution to the log-likelihood of a single unit with observed values (y, j, k) is

$$\log \mu_{jk}(\beta)^y (1 - \mu_{jk}(\beta))^{(1-y)} + \log \pi_{k|j} + \log \tau_j .$$

Hence maximization of the log-likelihood can be done independently for β, τ, and π, and the maximum likelihood (ML) estimate β_{ML}^{*n} of β results from maximizing

$$\ell_n^*(\beta) = \sum_{r=1}^n \ell^*(\beta; Y_r, X_{1r}, X_{2r})$$

with $\ell^*(\beta; y, j, k) := \log \mu_{jk}(\beta)^y (1 - \mu_{jk}(\beta))^{1-y}$.

β_{ML}^{*n} is consistent for the true parameter β^0 and asymptotically normal, i.e.

$$\sqrt{n}(\beta_{ML}^{*n} - \beta^0) \longrightarrow \mathcal{N}(0, I_{\beta\beta}^*(\beta^0, \pi^0, \tau^0)^{-1})$$

where π^0 and τ^0 are true parameter values and $I_{\beta\beta}^*(\beta, \pi, \tau)$ denotes the Fisher information matrix, i.e.,

$$I_{\beta\beta}^*(\beta, \pi, \tau) := - E_{\beta,\pi,\tau} \frac{\partial^2}{\partial\beta\partial\beta} \ell^*(\beta; Y, X_1, X_2)\Big|_\beta .$$

The computation of β_{ML}^{*n} involves an iterative method. We consider here the scoring-variant of the Newton Raphson method. The iterative step is given by

$$\beta^{t+1} = \beta^t + I_{\beta\beta}^*(\beta^t, \hat{\tau}^{*n}, \hat{\pi}^{*n})^{-1} S_n^*(\beta^t)$$

where $S_n^*(\beta)$ denotes the score function

$$S_n^*(\beta) := \frac{1}{n} \sum_{r=1}^n \frac{\partial}{\partial\beta} \ell^*(\beta; Y_r, X_{1r}, X_{2r})$$

and $\hat{\pi}^{*n}$ and $\hat{\tau}^{*n}$ are the ML estimates of π and τ, i.e.

$$\hat{\pi}_{k|j}^{*n} := \frac{n_{.jk}^*}{n_{.j.}^*} \quad \text{and} \quad \hat{\tau}_j^{*n} := \frac{n_{.j.}^*}{n} .$$

Estimation of the asymptotic variance can be based on the inverse of $I_{\beta\beta}^*(\beta_{ML}^{*n}, \hat{\pi}^{*n}, \hat{\tau}^{*n})$. Explicit representations of $I_{\beta\beta}^*(\beta, \pi, \tau)$ and $S_n^*(\beta)$ are given in Appendix B.1.

3. Missing Value Mechanisms

We now assume that we have missing values in the second covariate. The observability of X_2 is indicated by a random variable

$$O_2 := \begin{cases} 1 & \text{if } X_2 \text{ is observable} \\ 0 & \text{if } X_2 \text{ is unobservable} \end{cases} \qquad 2\dagger)$$

and instead of X_2 we observe the random variable

$$Z_2 := \begin{cases} X_2 & \text{if } O_2 = 1 \\ K+1 & \text{if } O_2 = 0 \end{cases}$$

with an additional category for missing values. Instead of $K+1$ we also use the symbol "?" for this category in the sequel.

The joint distribution of (Y, X_1, Z_2) depends on the conditional distribution of O_2 given (Y, X_1, X_2). This conditional distribution is called the *missing value mechanism*. The missing value mechanism is described by *the observation probabilities*

$$q_{ijk} := P(O_2 = 1 | Y = i, X_1 = j, X_2 = k). \tag{3.1}$$

Observing now n independent realizations $(Y_r, X_{1r}, Z_{2r})_{r=1,...,n}$ we have a $2 \times J \times (K+1)$ table with entries

$$n_{ijk} := \#\{r \mid Y_r = i, X_{1r} = j, Z_{2r} = k\}.$$

The cell probabilities for this table are

$$p_{ijk} := q_{ijk} p^*_{ijk} \text{ if } k \neq ? \qquad \text{and} \qquad p_{ij?} := \sum_{k=1}^{K} (1 - q_{ijk}) p^*_{ijk} ,$$

and with

$$q^A := \sum_{i=0}^{1} \sum_{j=1}^{J} p_{ij?}$$

we denote the *overall observation probability*. Without further restrictions on q_{ijk} the parameters β, π, τ and $q := (q_{ijk})_{i=0,1; j=1,...,J; k=1,...,K}$ are not identifiable. One assumption which allows identification excludes a dependence of the observation probability on the true value of the covariate, i.e., we assume

$$P(O_2 = 1 | Y = i, X_1 = j, X_2 = k) \equiv P(O_2 = 1 | Y = i, X_1 = j) =: q_{ij} .$$

2†) In the literature this variable is often denoted by R instead of O where R abbreviates *response*. As non-response is only one source of missing values, we prefer here the more general term *observability*. It may be more consequent to introduce a missing indicator M instead of an observability indicator O, but many formulas can be better expressed as functions of the observation probabilities than as functions of the missing probabilities.

This assumption is called *missing at random* (MAR) by Rubin (1976). It is fundamental for most statistical methods handling missing values in a sophisticated manner. From the practical point of view it is highly questionable in many applications. Not only the active refusal of an answer causes a violation of the MAR assumption, also the use of documents to collect covariate data is a source of such a violation. Often an event like a given therapy or an observed symptom is well documented, such that a gap in the documents is probable due to the absence of the event, because the latter is documented very seldom. In two of the examples mentioned in the introduction the MAR assumption is out of doubt: If we decide to add a new covariate during the recruitment of subjects in a prospective study, or if we restrict the collection of an expensive covariate to a subset of all subjects in advance. However, one should not overlook that the MAR assumption allows a dependence of the observation probabilities on the completely observed covariate and the outcome variable, i.e., it does not require that the units with a missing value are a random subsample. The latter is called the *missing completely at random* (MCAR) assumption, which requires

$$P(O_2 = 1 | Y = i, X_1 = j, X_2 = k) \equiv P(O_2 = 1) = q^A .$$

A typical example where it is important that we need not the MCAR assumption arises in case-control studies. Here the available sources for allocating information often differ between cases and controls and additionally an exposure variable like radiation treatment or occupational hazard is often associated with the availability of different documents, such that the probability of the occurrence of a missing values in a confounding variable depends on the outcome variable as well as on the exposure variable.

We now introduce two stronger restrictions than the MAR assumption, which reflect the asymmetry between the outcome variable Y and the covariate X_1. We consider the restrictions

$$P(O_2 = 1 | Y = i, X_1 = j) \equiv P(O_2 = 1 | X_1 = j)$$

which we call the *missing dependent on* X (MDX) assumption and

$$P(O_2 = 1 | Y = i, X_1 = j) \equiv P(O_2 = 1 | Y = i)$$

which we call the *missing dependent on* Y (MDY) assumption. Of course, MCAR implies MDX and MDY, and each of the latter implies MAR. We speak of an MDX missing value mechanism, if the MDX assumption is satisfied, but not the MCAR assumption, i.e. if the observation probabilities differ among the levels of X_1, but not among the levels of Y, and similar of an MDY mechanism. A MDXY missing value mechanism is a mechanism satisfying the MAR assumption but neither the MDX nor the MDY assumption. The situation of a case-control study described above is a typical example for an MDXY mechanism.

4. Estimation Methods

Methods to estimate the regression parameters of a logistic model in the presence of missing values in the covariates can be divided into two classes. The first class contains *ad-hoc-methods*, which try to manipulate the missing values in a simple manner in order to obtain an artificially completed table without missing values. The widespread use of these methods relates mainly to the fact that we can use standard statistical software for the analysis of the completed table. But a major drawback of these methods are their poor statistical properties. For many missing value mechanisms, even if they satisfy the MAR assumption, the methods may yield inconsistent estimates or they use the information of the incomplete observations in a very inefficient manner. Moreover the validity of variance estimates and confidence intervals is in doubt, because the process of manipulating the table is neglected. For the second class of methods consistency is implied by the estimation principle and estimates of asymptotic variance are available. The drawback of these methods is the increased effort for the implementation, because standard statistical software cannot be used directly.

We start our presentation with the three consistent estimation methods *Maximum Likelihood Estimation, Pseudo Maximum Likelihood Estimation*, and *Filling* which all belong to the second class. For these three methods we try to motivate their underlying ideas, state the main asymptotic properties and discuss the computation of estimates and the estimation of asymptotic variance. Subsequently we consider the ad-hoc methods *Complete Case Analysis, Probability Imputation, Additional Category* and *Omission of Covariate*. Here our presentation focuses on the source of bias implied by these methods, and a qualitative assessment of the magnitude of the bias is attempted by a comparison of the implicit modeling of these methods in contrast to the modeling of the pseudo maximum likelihood approach.

A quantitative assessment of the bias and a comparison of the efficiency of the consistent estimation methods is given in Chapters 5 and 6.

4.1 Maximum Likelihood Estimation

The Method

The applicability of the ML estimation principle also in the presence of missing values has been shown in a general manner by Rubin (1976). His basic result can be summarized in the following manner: If the MAR assumption holds, then for units with missing values in some variables ML estimation can be based on the marginal distribution omitting the unobserved variables (cf. Appendix A.1). In the sequel the ML estimation principle has been used in many fields of statistics to deal with missing values (Little & Rubin, 1987), but only very seldom for regression problems with missing values in the covariates. The reason is that the above given basic result can be only applied to the joint distribution of the variables, whereas in regression models the conditional distribution of the outcome variable is considered. But if one considers the joint distribution, then ML estimation of the regression parameters involves the additional estimation of nuisance parameters related to the distribution of the covariates, which is of course absolutely contrary to the complete data case.

These difficulties can be easily made evident in our special situation. The joint distribution of (Y, X_1, Z_2) is given by the cell probabilities

$$p_{ijk} = q_{ijk}\mu_{jk}(\beta)^i(1 - \mu_{jk}(\beta))^{1-i}\pi_{k|j}\tau_j \quad \text{for } k \neq ? \qquad \text{and}$$

$$p_{ij?} = \sum_{k=1}^{K}(1 - q_{ijk})\mu_{jk}(\beta)^i(1 - \mu_{jk}(\beta))^{1-i}\pi_{k|j}\tau_j \ . \tag{4.1}$$

The MAR assumption allows to factorize $p_{ij?}$ into

$$p_{ij?} = (1 - q_{ij})\left(\sum_{k=1}^{K}\mu_{jk}(\beta)^i(1 - \mu_{jk}(\beta))^{1-i}\pi_{k|j}\tau_j\right) \ .$$

Note that $\sum_{k=1}^{K}\mu_{jk}(\beta)^i(1 - \mu_{jk}(\beta))^{1-i}\pi_{k|j}\tau_j$ corresponds to the distribution of (Y, X_1), i.e., to the marginal distribution of observed variables. Using this factorization we can split the loglikelihood into three summands, one depending only on q, one depending only on τ, and one depending only on (β, π). But it is impossible to split the summand depending on (β, π) further, contrary to the complete data case (cf. Chapter 2). Hence ML estimation of β requires joint estimation of β and π, where we must regard π as a nuisance parameter.

The loglikelihood for (β, π) is now

$$\ell_{ML}^n(\beta, \pi) = \sum_{r=1}^{n}\ell^{ML}(\beta, \pi; Y_r, X_{1r}, Z_{2r})$$

with

$$\ell^{ML}(\beta, \pi; y, j, k) = \begin{cases} \log[\mu_{jk}(\beta)^y(1 - \mu_{jk}(\beta))^{1-y}] + \log\pi_{k|j} & \text{if } k \neq ? \\ \log[\sum_{k'=1}^{K}\mu_{jk'}(\beta)^y(1 - \mu_{jk'}(\beta))^{1-y}\pi_{k'|j}] & \text{if } k = ? \end{cases}$$

and the ML estimate $(\hat\beta_{ML}^n, \hat\pi_{ML}^n)$ maximizes this loglikelihood. [3†]

Asymptotic Distribution

To simplify the notation in the sequel, we introduce $\theta := (\beta, \pi)$ and $\xi := (\beta, \pi, \tau, q)$. With $\xi^0 = (\beta^0, \pi^0, \tau^0, q^0)$ we denote the true parameter vector.

Traditional theory yields consistency of $\hat\theta_{ML}^n$ for the true θ^0 and also the asymptotic normal distribution, where the covariance matrix is the inverse of the Fisher information matrix

$$I_{\theta\theta}^{ML}(\xi) = -E_\xi\frac{\partial^2}{\partial\theta\partial\theta}\ell^{ML}(\theta; Y, X_1, Z_2)\Big|_\xi$$

evaluated at ξ^0. As we are mainly interested in the covariance of $\hat\beta_{ML}^n$, we partition the Fisher information matrix into

$$\begin{pmatrix} I_{\beta\beta}^{ML}(\xi) & I_{\beta\pi}^{ML}(\xi) \\ I_{\beta\pi}^{ML}(\xi)' & I_{\pi\pi}^{ML}(\xi) \end{pmatrix}$$

and we have

$$\sqrt{n}(\hat\beta_{ML}^n - \beta^0) \rightarrow \mathcal{N}(0, [I_{\beta\beta}^{ML}(\xi^0) - I_{\beta\pi}^{ML}(\xi^0)I_{\pi\pi}^{ML}(\xi^0)^{-1}I_{\beta\pi}^{ML}(\xi^0)']^{-1}) \ . \tag{4.2}$$

[3†] It is an open question, whether the loglikelihood $\ell_{ML}^n(\beta, \pi)$ is unimodal or not. It can be easily shown that the function is not convex, but in spite of some efforts no example could be found, where we have really two local maxima.

Computation of Estimates

For the maximization of the loglikelihood two basically different algorithms are available: The expectation maximization (EM) algorithm and the Newton-Raphson method or one of its variants. For the scoring-variant of the Newton-Raphson method the iteration step is

$$\theta^{t+1} = \theta^t + I_{\theta\theta}^{ML}(\theta^t, \hat{\tau}^n, \hat{q}^n) S_{ML}^n(\theta^t)$$

where

$$S_{ML}^n(\theta) := \frac{1}{n} \sum_{r=1}^N \frac{\partial}{\partial\theta} \ell^{ML}(\theta; Y_r, X_{1r}, Z_{2r})\Big|_\theta$$

is the score function, and $\hat{\tau}^n$ and $\hat{q}^n$ are the ML estimates given by

$$\hat{\tau}_j^n := \frac{n_{.j.}}{n} \quad \text{and} \quad \hat{q}_{ij}^n := \frac{n_{ij+}}{n_{ij.}} \quad \text{with} \quad n_{ij+} := \sum_{k=1}^K n_{ijk} \ .$$

Explicit representations of $I_{\theta\theta}^{ML}(\xi)$ and $S_{ML}^n(\theta)$ are given in Appendix B.2.

The EM algorithm is a general tool to maximize a likelihood arising in a missing value problem. A general description is given in Appendix A.2. In our problem the EM algorithm yields the following simple form: Given the values (β^t, π^t) of the t-th step, in the E-step a new $2 \times J \times K$ contingency table n^{t+1} is constructed with entries

$$n_{ijk}^{t+1} := n_{ijk} + n_{ij?} \, r_{k|ij}(\beta^t, \pi^t)$$

$$\text{with} \quad r_{k|ij}(\beta, \pi) := P_{\beta,\pi}(X_2 = k | Y = i, X_1 = j) = \frac{\pi_{k|j}\mu_{jk}(\beta)^i(1 - \mu_{jk}(\beta))^{1-i}}{\sum_{k'=1}^K \pi_{k'|j}\mu_{jk'}(\beta)^i(1 - \mu_{jk'}(\beta))^{1-i}} \ .$$

In the M-step β^{t+1} is received by computing the ML estimate of β from the complete table n^{t+1}. π^{t+1} is the ML estimate of π from this table, i.e.,

$$\pi_{k|j}^{t+1} := \frac{n_{.jk}^{t+1}}{n_{.j.}} \ .$$

Estimation of Asymptotic Variance

If we evaluate the Fisher information $I_{\theta\theta}^{ML}(\xi)$ at $\hat{\xi}^n = (\hat{\beta}_{ML}^n, \hat{\pi}_{ML}^n, \hat{\tau}^n, \hat{q}^n)$, then $\frac{1}{n}I_{\theta\theta}^{ML}(\hat{\xi}^n)^{-1}$ is an estimate of the covariance of $\hat{\theta}_{ML}^n$.

The computation of $I_{\theta\theta}^{ML}(\hat{\xi}^n)$ can be based on explicit formulas given in Appendix B.2. Especially if the EM algorithm is used for the solution of the maximization task, it suggests itself to use a representation of $I_{\theta\theta}^{ML}$ relating it to the Fisher information and the score function of the complete data case. Such a relation has been shown by Louis (1982), cf. Appendix A.2.

Based on

$$-\frac{\partial^2}{\partial\theta\partial\theta} \ell^{ML}(\theta; y, j, k)\Big|_\theta$$

$$= E_{\theta,\tau,q}\left[-\frac{\partial^2}{\partial\theta\partial\theta}\ell^*(\theta; y, j, X_2)\big|_{\theta} \,\Big|\, Y = y, X_1 = j, Z_2 = k \right]$$

$$- Var_{\theta,\tau,q}\left[\frac{\partial}{\partial\theta}\ell^*(\theta; y, j, X_2)\big|_{\theta} \,\Big|\, Y = y, X_1 = j, Z_2 = k \right]$$

with $\ell^*(\theta; y, j, k) = \ell^*(\beta; y, j, k) + \log \pi_{k|j}$ denoting the loglikelihood for the joint estimation of β and π in the complete data case, we have

$$I_{\theta\theta}^{ML}(\xi) = I_{\theta\theta}^*(\xi) - E_\xi H_{\theta\theta}(Y, X_1, Z_2) \tag{4.3}$$

with $H_{\theta\theta}(y, j, k) := Var\left[\frac{\partial}{\partial\theta}\ell^*(\theta; y, j, X_2)\big|_{\theta} \,\Big|\, Y = y, X_1 = j, Z_2 = k \right]$.

Here $I_{\theta\theta}^*(\xi)$ is the Fisher information of the joint estimation of β and π in the complete data case. $I_{\theta\theta}^*(\xi)$ is a block diagonal matrix with the blocks $I_{\beta\beta}^*(\xi)$ and $I_{\pi\pi}^*(\xi)$. Further we have $H_{\theta\theta}(y, j, k) = 0$ if $k \neq ?$, and hence

$$E_\xi H_{\theta\theta}(Y, X_1, Z_2)$$

$$= \sum_{j=1}^{J} H_{\theta\theta}(1, j, ?) P_\xi(Y = 1, X_1 = j, Z_2 = ?) + H_{\theta\theta}(0, j, ?) P_\xi(Y = 0, X_1 = j, Z_2 = ?)$$

$$= \sum_{j=1}^{J} [H_{\theta\theta}(1, j, ?)(1 - q_{1j})\mu_{j?}(\beta, \pi) + H_{\theta\theta}(0, j, ?)(1 - q_{0j})(1 - \mu_{j?}(\beta, \pi))] \tau_j .$$

Explicit representations of $I_{\pi\pi}^*(\xi)$, $\frac{\partial}{\partial\theta}\ell^*(\theta; y, j, k)$, and $H_{\theta\theta}(y, j, ?)$ are given in Appendix B.1 and B.2, respectively. Using standard statistical software for the maximization task of the M-step, we may receive from the last step an estimate of $I_{\beta\beta}^*(\xi^0)$ or at least its inverse. The other quantities $I_{\pi\pi}^*(\xi)$ and $E_\xi H_{\theta\theta}(Y, X_1, Z_2)$ have to be evaluated at $\hat{\xi}^n$.

References

A first suggestion to handle the problem of missing covariate data in a logistic regression model via ML estimation can be found in Little & Schluchter (1985). ML estimation in the general class of generalized linear models with categorical covariates is considered by Ibrahim (1990), so that the results here are a special case. Using the relation between logistic regression and loglinear models, some results can be also found in Fuchs (1982).

4.2 Pseudo Maximum Likelihood Estimation

The Method

In the last section we have started our considerations from the point of view of a general estimation principle. Here we start with the idea to look at the problem from the point of view of regression models, i.e., to consider the conditional distribution of the outcome variable Y given the covariates X_1 and Z_2.

For this conditional distribution we find for $k \neq ?$

$$P(Y = 1|X_1 = j, Z_2 = k)$$

$$= \frac{P(Y = 1, X_1 = j, X_2 = k, O_2 = 1)}{P(X_1 = j, X_2 = k, O_2 = 1)}$$

$$= \frac{P(O_2 = 1|Y = 1, X_1 = j, X_2 = k)P(Y = 1, X_1 = j, X_2 = k)}{P(O_2 = 1|X_1 = j, X_2 = k)P(X_1 = j, X_2 = k)}$$

$$= \frac{q_{1jk}}{q_{1jk}\mu_{jk}(\beta) + q_{0jk}(1 - \mu_{jk}(\beta))}\mu_{jk}(\beta)$$

and

$$P(Y = 1|X_1 = j, Z_2 =?)$$

$$= \frac{P(Y = 1, X_1 = j, O_2 = 0)}{P(X_1 = j, O_2 = 0)}$$

$$= \frac{P(O_2 = 0|Y = 1, X_1 = j)P(Y = 1, X_1 = j)}{P(O_2 = 0|X_1 = j)P(X_1 = j)}$$

$$= \frac{\sum_{k=1}^{K} P(O_2 = 0|Y = 1, X_1 = j, X_2 = k)P(X_2 = k|Y = 1, X_1 = j)}{\sum_{k=1}^{K} P(O_2 = 0|X_1 = j, X_2 = k)P(X_2 = k|X_1 = j)}P(Y = 1|X_1 = j)$$

$$= \frac{\sum_{k=1}^{K} P(O_2 = 0|Y = 1, X_1 = j, X_2 = k)P(X_2 = k|Y = 1, X_1 = j)}{\sum_{k=1}^{K}\left[\sum_{i=0}^{1}P(O_2=0|Y=i, X_1=j, X_2=k)P(Y=i|X_1=j, X_2=k)\right]P(X_2=k|X_1=j)}$$

$$\times \sum_{k=1}^{K} P(Y = 1|X_1 = j, X_2 = k)P(X_2 = k|X_1 = j)$$

$$= \frac{\sum_{k=1}^{K}(1 - q_{1jk})r_{k|ij}(\beta, \pi)}{\sum_{k=1}^{K}\left[(1 - q_{0jk})(1 - \mu_{jk}(\beta)) + (1 - q_{1jk})\mu_{jk}(\beta)\right]\pi_{k|j}}\mu_{j?}(\beta, \pi)$$

with $\mu_{j?}(\beta, \pi) = \sum_{k=1}^{K}\pi_{k|j}\Lambda(\beta_0 + \beta_{1j} + \beta_{2k})$.

If we now assume not only MAR but make the stronger MDX assumption, i.e., we exclude a dependence of the observability of X_2 on the true value of X_2 and on the outcome variable, then the factors in front of $\mu_{jk}(\beta)$ and $\mu_{j?}(\beta, \pi)$ disappear, and we have

$$P(Y = 1 | X_1 = j, Z_2 = k) = \mu_{jk}(\beta) \quad \text{if } k \neq ? \quad \text{and}$$
$$P(Y = 1 | X_1 = j, Z_2 = ?) = \mu_{j?}(\beta, \pi) . \tag{4.4}$$

Again the nuisance parameter π appears. But under the MDX assumption it is straightforward to estimate π by

$$\hat{\pi}_{k|j}^n := \frac{n_{.jk}}{n_{.j+}} \tag{4.5}$$

which is a consistent estimate. Taking this estimate as the true value of π, we arrive from (4.4) at the loglikelihood

$$\ell_{PML}^n(\beta) = \sum_{r=1}^{n} \ell^{PML}(\beta, \hat{\pi}^n; Y_r, X_{1r}, Z_{2r})$$

with

$$\ell^{PML}(\beta, \pi; y, j, k) = \begin{cases} \log[\mu_{jk}(\beta)^y (1 - \mu_{jk}(\beta))^{1-y}] & \text{if } k \neq ? \\ \log[\mu_{j?}(\beta, \pi)^y (1 - \mu_{j?}(\beta, \pi))^{1-y}] & \text{if } k = ? \end{cases} .$$

With

$$m^n(\pi) := \sum_{r=1}^{n} m(\pi; X_{1r}, Z_{2r}) \text{ and } m(\pi; j, k) = \begin{cases} \log \pi_{k|j} & \text{if } k \neq ? \\ 0 & \text{if } k = ? \end{cases}$$

we have

$$\ell_{PML}^n(\beta) = \ell_{ML}^n(\beta, \hat{\pi}^n) - m^n(\hat{\pi}^n) ;$$

hence considering ℓ_{PML}^n instead of ℓ_{ML}^n means to replace π in the loglikelihood of the joint estimation of β and π by a consistent estimate. The effect of substituting parameters in a loglikelihood by estimates has been considered by several authors (Gong & Samaniego 1981, Pierce 1982, Randles 1982, Parke 1986). According to Gong & Samaniego (1981) we call $\hat{\beta}_{PML}^n$ maximizing ℓ_{PML}^n a pseudo maximum likelihood estimate.

The conditional distributions considered above are more complex if we consider the weaker MAR assumption. But from the view of pseudo maximum likelihood estimation it suffices to substitute π in ℓ_{ML}^n by a consistent estimate. $\hat{\pi}^n$ defined in (4.5) is not necessarily consistent assuming MAR. An estimate $\tilde{\pi}^n$ which is always consistent [4†] assuming MAR is given by

$$\tilde{\pi}_{k|j}^n := \frac{n_{0j.} \frac{n_{0jk}}{n_{0j+}} + n_{1j.} \frac{n_{1jk}}{n_{1j+}}}{n_{0j.} + n_{1j.}} ; \tag{4.6}$$

hence we have just to consider $\ell_{ML}^n(\beta, \tilde{\pi}^n)$ as the pseudo loglikelihood, and we receive the

---

[4†] Consistency can be easily seen by the fact that $\tilde{\pi}^n$ is just the estimate $\hat{\pi}^{*n}$ applied to a contingency table with consistent estimates of the true cell probabilities, which we will introduce in Section 4.3.

alternative estimate $\check{\beta}^n_{PML}$ by maximizing over β. If we come back to the view from the conditional distributions, the loglikelihood would depend on the additional parameter q, and we can decompose it into

$$\ell^n(\beta, \tau, q) = \ell^n_{ML}(\beta, \pi) - m^n(\pi) + h^n(\beta, \pi, q) \, .$$

$\ell^n_{PML}(\beta)$ neglects the last term, hence we also can regard $\check{\beta}^n_{PML}$ as a pseudo partial likelihood estimate.

Asymptotic Distribution

It is well known that substituting some parameters in a likelihood by consistent estimates and maximizing over the remaining parameters does not destroy consistency and asymptotic normality (Gong & Samaniego 1981). Only the asymptotic variance becomes somewhat more complex than the inversion of the information matrix, because we have to adjust for the additional variance caused by the inefficient estimation of the substituted parameters.

Let $\check{\pi}^n$ denote an arbitrary consistent estimate for π and $\check{\beta}^n_{PML}$ should be a root of $\frac{\partial}{\partial \beta} \ell^n_{ML}(\beta, \check{\pi}^n)$. Taylor expansion of the score function about β^0 yields

$$I^{ML}_{\beta\beta}(\xi^0)\sqrt{n}(\check{\beta}^n_{PML} - \beta^0) = n^{-\frac{1}{2}} \frac{\partial}{\partial \beta} \ell^n_{ML}(\beta^0, \check{\pi}^n) + o_p(1) \tag{4.7}$$

and a second expansion of $\ell^n_{ML}(\beta^0, \check{\pi}^n)$ about π^0 results in

$$I^{ML}_{\beta\beta}(\xi^0)\sqrt{n}(\check{\beta}^n_{PML} - \beta^0) = n^{-\frac{1}{2}} \frac{\partial}{\partial \beta} \ell^n_{ML}(\beta^0, \pi^0) - I^{ML}_{\beta\pi}(\xi^0)\sqrt{n}(\check{\pi}^n - \pi^0) + o_p(1) \tag{4.8}$$

where the remainders can be examined by extending the proof of Gong & Samaniego (1981) to the multiparameter case using for example the technique of Lehmann (1983), p. 430. Now $n^{-\frac{1}{2}} \frac{\partial}{\partial \beta} \ell^n_{ML}(\beta^0, \pi^0)$ is asymptotically normal with mean 0 and variance $I^{ML}_{\beta\beta}(\xi^0)$. If $n^{-\frac{1}{2}} \frac{\partial}{\partial \beta} \ell^n_{ML}(\beta^0, \pi^0)$ and $\sqrt{n}(\check{\pi}^n - \pi^0)$ are asymptotically independent, then the asymptotic variance of $\sqrt{n}(\check{\beta}^n_{PML} - \beta^0)$ is

$$I^{ML}_{\beta\beta}(\xi^0)^{-1} + I^{ML}_{\beta\beta}(\xi^0)^{-1} I^{ML}_{\beta\pi}(\xi^0)\Sigma_{\check{\pi}^n}(\xi^0)I^{ML}_{\beta\pi}(\xi^0)' I^{ML}_{\beta\beta}(\xi^0)^{-1} \tag{4.9}$$

with $\Sigma_{\check{\pi}^n}(\xi^0)$ denoting the asymptotic variance of $\sqrt{n}(\check{\pi}^n - \pi^0)$. Note that we can write the asymptotic variance (4.2) of the ML estimate similar as

$$I^{ML}_{\beta\beta}(\xi^0)^{-1} + I^{ML}_{\beta\beta}(\xi^0)^{-1} I^{ML}_{\beta\pi}(\xi^0)\Sigma_{\hat{\pi}^n_{ML}}(\xi^0)I^{ML}_{\beta\pi}(\xi^0)' I^{ML}_{\beta\beta}(\xi^0)^{-1} \tag{4.10}$$

demonstrating that we have just to change the variance of the nuisance parameters estimate. As $I^{ML}_{\beta\beta}(\xi^0)^{-1}$ denotes the variance of the maximum likelihood estimate of β if π is known, the additional terms can be regarded as the necessary correction due to the fact that π is estimated.

The asymptotic independence of $n^{-\frac{1}{2}} \frac{\partial}{\partial \beta} \ell^n_{ML}(\beta^0, \pi^0)$ and $\sqrt{n}(\hat{\pi}^n - \pi^0)$ for $\hat{\pi}^n$ given by (4.5) can be easily established: $\hat{\pi}^n$ results from minimizing $m^n(\pi)$, hence $\sqrt{n}(\hat{\pi}^n - \pi^0)$ is asymptotically equivalent to a linear transformation of $n^{-\frac{1}{2}} \frac{\partial}{\partial \pi} m^n(\pi^0)$, and $E\left(\frac{\partial}{\partial \beta} \ell^{ML}(\beta^0, \pi^0; Y, X_1, Z_2)\frac{\partial}{\partial \pi} m(\pi^0, X_1, Z_2)\right) = 0$ holds, because we have

$E\left[\frac{\partial}{\partial\beta}\ell^{ML}(\beta^0,\pi^0;Y,X_1,Z_2)\Big|X_1,Z_2\right] = 0$. Hence the asymptotic variance of $\hat{\beta}^n_{PML}$ is given by (4.9).

Unfortunately $\tilde{\pi}^n$ given by (4.6) and $n^{-\frac{1}{2}}\frac{\partial}{\partial\beta}\ell^n_{ML}(\beta^0,\pi^0)$ are not asymptotically independent, as the weights $n_{ij.}/n_{.j.}$ are correlated with the estimates for β_{1j} if π is known. To achieve an explicit representation for the asymptotic variance from (4.8) we need an explicit representation for the covariance, which is burdensome to achieve. A simpler way is to regard $n^{-1}\frac{\partial}{\partial\beta}\ell^n_{ML}(\beta^0,\tilde{\pi}^n)$ as a function $g_\beta(\beta^0,\hat{p}^n)$ of the relative cell frequencies $\hat{p}^n := (\hat{p}^n_{ijk})_{i=0,1;j=1,\dots,J;k=1,\dots,K+1}$ with $\hat{p}^n_{ijk} := n_{ijk}/n$. The delta method allows to represent the asymptotic variance of $n^{-\frac{1}{2}}\frac{\partial}{\partial\beta}\ell^n_{ML}(\beta^0,\tilde{\pi}^n)$ as $J_{\beta p}(\xi^0)\Sigma_{\hat{p}^n}J_{\beta p}(\xi^0)'$ where $J_{\beta p}(\xi^0) := \frac{\partial}{\partial p}g_\beta(\beta^0,p)\big|_{p^0}$ and Σ^n_p is the asymptotic covariance of $\sqrt{n}(\hat{p}^n - p^0)$. Using (4.7) the asymptotic covariance of $\sqrt{n}(\hat{\beta}^n_{PML} - \beta^0)$ is hence

$$I^{ML}_{\beta\beta}(\xi^0)^{-1}J_{\beta p}(\xi^0)\Sigma_{\hat{p}^n}J_{\beta p}(\xi^0)'I^{ML}_{\beta\beta}(\xi^0)^{-1} . \tag{4.11}$$

Explicit representations for $J_{\beta p}(\xi^0)$ and $\Sigma_{\hat{p}^n}$ are given in Appendix B.3.

It remains the interesting question, whether there exists a simple estimate $\tilde{\pi}^n$ for π, which is always consistent and asymptotically independent from $n^{-\frac{1}{2}}\frac{\partial}{\partial\beta}\ell^n_{ML}(\beta^0,\pi^0)$. A nonsimple estimate with this property exists: the maximum likelihood estimate, which follows implicitly from the variance representations (4.9) and (4.10). This asymptotic independence can be also established by asymptotic efficiency (Pierce 1982).

Computation of Estimates

As in the computation of the ML estimates we can use the EM algorithm or a Newton-Raphson method to compute the estimates. In the scoring variant of the Newton-Raphson method the iteration step is given by

$$\beta^{t+1} = \beta^t + I^{ML}_{\beta\beta}(\beta^t,\check{\pi}^n,\hat{\tau}^n,\hat{q}^n)S^n_{PML}(\beta^t,\check{\pi}^n)$$

where $S^n_{PML}(\beta,\pi)$ is just $S^n_{ML}(\beta,\pi)$ restricted to the derivates with respect to β, and $\check{\pi}^n$ is either $\hat{\pi}^n$ or $\tilde{\pi}^n$. This algorithm can be also expressed as an iterated weighted linear regression, which follows from the results of Wedderburn (1974); cf. also Thompson & Baker (1981).

Using the EM algorithm, the procedure is similar to that of ML Estimation. We have just to replace $r_{k|ij}(\beta^t,\pi^t)$ by $r_{k|ij}(\beta^t,\check{\pi}^n)$, and the computation of π^t is dropped.

Estimation of Asymptotic Variance

For the estimation of the asymptotic variance of $\hat{\beta}^n_{PML}$ or $\tilde{\beta}^n_{PML}$ we have to evaluate the quantities in (4.9) or (4.11), respectively, at $\hat{\xi}^n_{PML} := (\hat{\beta}^n_{PML},\check{\pi}^n,\hat{\tau}^n,\hat{q}^n)$ or $\tilde{\xi}^n_{PML} := (\tilde{\beta}^n_{PML},\check{\pi}^n,\hat{\tau}^n,\hat{q}^n)$, respectively.

References

Pepe & Fleming (1991) consider this technique under the MDX assumption, but in a more general framework allowing also that X_2 is continuous. Hence they use also another technique to estimate the asymptotic variance. The extension to MDY and MDXY missing value mechanisms is shown in Vach & Schumacher (1992, 1993). Maximum Likelihood estimation with known π is considered by Whittemore & Grosser (1986).

4.3 The Filling Method

The Method

A straightforward idea is the following two-step procedure: We first try to reconstruct the true, but unobservable table $(n_{ijk}^*)_{i=0,1;j=1,...,J;k=1,...,K}$ and then we apply a logistic regression to the reconstructed table. In the first step we have to distribute the units $n_{ij?}$ to the cells (i,j,k) with $k = 1,\dots,K$. The fraction of $n_{ij?}$ distributed to the cell (i,j,k) should be proportional to the probability that k is the true value of X_2. Estimating this probability by $\frac{n_{ijk}}{n_{ij+}}$, the "filled" table is

$$\hat{n}_{ijk}^* := n_{ijk} + n_{ij?}\frac{n_{ijk}}{n_{ij+}} \ .$$

From this table we yield the estimate $\hat{\beta}_{FILL}^n$ by applying a logistic regression as in the complete data case.

Asymptotic Distribution

The relative cell frequencies

$$\hat{\hat{p}}^{*n} := \frac{\hat{n}_{ijk}^*}{n} \ ^{5\dagger)}$$

of the filled table are the ML estimates of the true cell probabilities p_{ijk}^* under a multinomial model and assuming MAR (cf. Little & Rubin 1987, p. 173). Hence they are consistent. The complete data estimates of a logistic regression continuously depend on the relative cell frequencies, hence $\hat{\beta}_{FILL}^n$ is consistent for β.

To achieve the asymptotic distribution of $\hat{\beta}_{FILL}^n$, we have to look at the estimation equations solved by $\hat{\beta}_{FILL}^n$. They are given by

$$S(\beta, \hat{\hat{p}}^{*n}) = 0$$

$$\text{with } S(\beta, p^*) := \sum_{j=1}^{J}\sum_{k=1}^{K} p_{1jk}^* \frac{\partial}{\partial\beta}\log\Lambda(\beta_0+\beta_{1j}+\beta_{2k}) + p_{0jk}^*\frac{\partial}{\partial\beta}\log[1-\Lambda(\beta_0+\beta_{1j}+\beta_{2k})]$$

where $S(\beta,\hat{\hat{p}}^{*n})$ can be regarded as an estimate for the true score function $S_n^*(\beta)$. A Taylor expansion of $S(\beta,\hat{\hat{p}}^{*n})$ about β^0 yields as in the complete data case

$$I_{\beta\beta}^*(\xi^0)\sqrt{n}(\hat{\beta}_{FILL}^n - \beta^0) = \sqrt{n}S(\beta^0,\hat{\hat{p}}^{*n}) + o_p(1) \ .$$

A second Taylor expansion of $S(\beta,p^*)$ at p^{*0} yields

$$\sqrt{n}S(\beta,\hat{\hat{p}}^{*n}) = H_{\beta p^*}(\beta^0, p^{*0})\sqrt{n}(\hat{\hat{p}}^{*n} - p^{*0}) + o_p(1)$$

$^{5\dagger)}$ The double hat should emphasize that these are estimates for the unobservable estimates $\hat{p}_{ijk}^{*n} := \frac{n_{ijk}^*}{n}$

with $H_{\beta p*}(\beta, p^*) := \dfrac{\partial}{\partial p^*} S(\beta, p^*)\big|_{\beta, p^*}$.

Hence

$$\sqrt{n}(\hat{\beta}^n_{FILL} - \beta^0) \tag{4.12}$$

$$\rightarrow \mathcal{N}(0, I^*_{\beta\beta}(\xi^0)^{-1} H_{\beta p*}(\beta^0, p^{*0}) \Sigma_{\hat{p}^{*n}}(\xi^0) H_{\beta p*}(\beta^0, p^{*0})' I^*_{\beta\beta}(\xi^0)^{-1})$$

where $\Sigma_{\hat{p}^{*n}}(\xi^0)$ is the asymptotic variance of of $\sqrt{n}(\hat{\bar{p}}^{*n} - p^{*0})$. As $\hat{\bar{p}}^{*n}$ is a function of the observed cell frequencies $\hat{p}^n$, an explicit representation of $\Sigma_{\hat{p}^{*n}}(\xi^0)$ can be achieved using the delta method. This and an explicit representation of $H_{\beta p*}$ are given in Appendix B.4.

The above arguments of establishing asymptotic normality and finding a representation of the asymptotic variance have been studied in a more general framework by Benichou & Gail (1989).

Computation of Estimates

Computation of $\hat{\beta}^n_{FILL}$ can be done with standard statistical software for logistic regression, just by applying the procedure to the table $(\hat{n}^*_{ijk})_{i=0,1;j=1,...,J;k=1,...,K}$. If the software does not allow the use of fractional values for the cell entries, it is possible to multiply the cell entries with a large number to achieve approximate integer values. Such a multiplication does not change the estimate.

Estimation of Asymptotic Variance

The quantities in (4.12) are evaluated at $\hat{\xi}^n_{FILL} := (\hat{\beta}^n_{FILL}, \tilde{\pi}^n, \hat{\tau}^n, \hat{q}^n)$ where $\tilde{\pi}^n$ is just the estimate $\hat{\pi}^{*n}$ applied to the filled table. Note that $H_{\beta p*}(\beta, p^*)$ does not depend on p^* (as shown in Appendix B.4).

The explicit computation of $I^*_{\beta\beta}(\hat{\xi}^n_{FILL})^{-1}$ can be avoided, because this is an estimate of the asymptotic variance of the complete data estimates, and such an estimate is also provided by statistical standard software applied to the filled table $(\hat{n}^*_{ijk})_{i=0,1;j=1,...,J;k=1,...,K}$. Hence (4.12) is also a formula how to correct this wrong variance estimate, but unfortunately this correction cannot be expressed as a simple rule like adding something to the wrong estimate.

Relation to ML Estimation

From the general theory of ML estimation in the presence of missing values it is well known that

$$S^n_{ML}(\beta, \pi) = E_{\beta, \pi}\left[S^*_n(\beta)\big|(n_{ijk})_{i=0,1;j=1,...,J;k=1,...,K+1}\right] ,$$

i.e., the score function is just the expectation of the true score function given the observed data (cf. Tanner 1991, p. 37). As $S^*_n(\beta)$ is linear in $\hat{p}^{*n}$, we have

$$S^n_{ML}(\beta, \pi) = S\left(\beta, E_{\beta, \pi}\left[\hat{p}^{*n}\big|(n_{ijk})_{i=0,1;j=1,...,J;k=1,...,K+1}\right]\right)$$

where $\hat{p}^{*n}$ are the true, but unobserved relative cell frequencies. Now

$$E_{\beta,\pi}\left[\hat{p}_{ijk}^{*n}\,\Big|\,(n_{ijk})_{i=0,1;j=1,\dots,J;k=1,\dots,K+1}\right]$$

$$= n_{ijk} + P_{\beta,\pi}(X_2 = k|Y=i, X_1 = j)n_{ij?} = n_{ijk} + r_{k|ij}(\beta,\pi)n_{ij?}$$

holds. In the score function of the Filling method $r_{k|ij}(\beta,\pi)$ is replaced by $\frac{n_{ijk}}{n_{ij+}}$, i.e. by a non-parametric estimate neglecting the dependence on the regression parameters.

This similarity between ML Estimation and the Filling approach is also visible in the algorithms to compute the estimates. The Filling method is just one step of the EM algorithm with the same substitution as above, cf. Section 4.1.

Filling as Weighting

The Filling method can be also regarded as a weighting approach. We have

$$\hat{n}_{ijk}^* = n_{ijk}\left(1 + \frac{n_{ij?}}{n_{ij+}}\right) = \frac{n_{ijk}}{\hat{q}_{ij}^n} \qquad \text{with } \hat{q}_{ij}^n := \frac{n_{ij+}}{n_{ij\cdot}}$$

such that $\hat{q}_{ij}^n$ are estimates for the observation probabilities. Hence each cell of the contingency table $(n_{ijk})_{i=0,1;j=1,\dots,J;k=1,\dots,K}$ is just weighted reciprocally to its observation probability. Such an approach is well known in survey sampling theory generalizing the Horvitz-Thompson estimate of a population quantity (Oh & Scheuren 1983). But here the idea is applied to the score function.

References

The Filling method was first proposed by Vach & Blettner (1991), but without deriving the asymptotic distribution. The idea to weight the contributions to the score function reciprocally to the observation probability is also used by Flanders & Greenland (1991) and Zhao & Lipsitz (1992). However, they consider the analysis of designs, where the observation probabilities are known. Wild (1991) considers a similar technique for the analysis of retrospective studies with completely missing covariate information for some units. Filling is a special case of the Mean Score Method proposed by Reilly (1991) and Reilly & Pepe (1993a).

It is worth mentioning that Filling cannot be regarded as an imputation technique, because we do not impute single guesses for the missing values.

4.4 Complete Case Analysis

The Method

In a Complete Case Analysis the data is restricted to units with complete information on X_2.

Asymptotic Bias

If we restrict our data to units with complete information, the correct modeling for the remaining units is

$$P(Y=1|X_1=j, Z_2=k) = \frac{q_{ijk}}{q_{0jk}(1-\mu_{jk}(\beta)) + q_{1jk}(1-\mu_{jk}(\beta))}\mu_{jk}(\beta),$$

cf. Section 4.2. But the Complete Case Analysis is based on the modeling

$$P(Y = 1|X_1 = j, Z_2 = k) = \mu_{jk}(\beta).$$

This modeling coincides with the true one, if and only if $q_{ijk} \equiv q_{jk}$, i.e., if the probability for the occurrence of a missing value does not depend on the outcome variable. Hence under this assumption the Complete Case Analysis yields consistent estimates and asymptotically valid confidence intervals.

It remains the question what happens if $q_{ijk} \neq q_{jk}$. In order to give an answer we consider the odds ratios within the units with complete information on X_2. For the cell probabilities of the contingency table built by these units we find

$$p_{ijk}^{CC} := P(Y = i, X_1 = j, X_2 = k|O_2 = 1)$$

$$= \frac{P(O_2 = 1|Y = i, X_1 = j, X_2 = k)P(Y = i, X_1 = j, X_2 = k)}{P(O_2 = 1)}$$

$$= \frac{q_{ijk}p_{ijk}^*}{q^A};$$

hence the odds ratio between the j-th category of X_1 and the first one given $X_2 = k$ is

$$\phi_{jk}^{CC} := \frac{p_{1jk}^* p_{01k}^*}{p_{0jk}^* p_{11k}^*} \frac{q_{1jk}q_{01k}}{q_{0jk}q_{11k}} = \phi_j^* Q_{jk}^\phi \quad \text{with } Q_{jk}^\phi := \frac{q_{1jk}q_{01k}}{q_{0jk}q_{11k}}$$

and the odds ratio between the k-th category of X_2 and the first one given $X_1 = j$ is

$$\psi_{jk}^{CC} := \frac{p_{1jk}^* p_{0j1}^*}{p_{0jk}^* p_{1j1}^*} \frac{q_{1jk}q_{0j1}}{q_{0jk}q_{1j1}} = \psi_k^* Q_{jk}^\psi \quad \text{with } Q_{jk}^\psi := \frac{q_{1jk}q_{0j1}}{q_{0jk}q_{1j1}}$$

where ϕ_j^* and ψ_k^* are the true odds ratios. Now if $Q_{jk}^\phi = 1$ and $Q_{jk}^\psi = 1$ then the odds ratios of the units with complete information on X_2 are equal to the true ones, and hence applying a logistic regression yields consistent estimates. The following table lists the values of Q_{jk}^ϕ and Q_{jk}^ψ for different assumptions on q_{ijk}:

	Q_{jk}^ϕ	Q_{jk}^ψ
$q_{ijk} \equiv q_{jk}$	1	1
$q_{ijk} \equiv q_i$	1	1
$q_{ijk} \equiv q_{ij}$	$\frac{q_{1j}q_{01}}{q_{0j}q_{11}}$	1
$q_{ijk} \equiv q_{ik}$	1	$\frac{q_{1k}q_{01}}{q_{0k}q_{11}}$

Besides the assumption $q_{ijk} \equiv q_{jk}$ mentioned above also the assumption $q_{ijk} \equiv q_i$ implies consistent estimation of odds ratios. This corresponds to the justification of logistic regression models in the analysis of case-control studies: If the selection probabilities depend only on the outcome variable then in an underlying logistic model only the intercept changes. In all other situations, consistent estimation cannot be warranted. In the most general case, where

q_{ijk} really depends on all three indices, the odds ratios of the units with complete information are not constant, and it is not obvious, to which values the estimates of the Complete Case Analysis converge. But if $q_{ijk} \equiv q_{ij}$ or $q_{ijk} \equiv q_{ik}$ then the odds ratios are constant and hence the Complete Case Analysis yields consistent estimates of these odds ratios and the bias ratio is equal to Q_{jk}^{ϕ} or Q_{jk}^{ψ}, respectively. For example under the MAR assumption $q_{ijk} \equiv q_{ij}$ the bias ratio in estimating ϕ_j by a complete case analysis is $\frac{q_{1j}q_{01}}{q_{0j}q_{11}}$. This bias ratio can be larger or smaller than 1.0, i.e., underestimation as well as overestimation can occur. Looking at some possible values of the bias ratio in the following table

q_{01}	q_{0j}	q_{11}	q_{1j}	$\frac{q_{1j}q_{01}}{q_{0j}q_{11}}$
0.6	0.8	0.7	0.9	0.96
0.6	0.9	0.7	0.8	0.76
0.7	0.8	0.6	0.9	1.31
0.5	0.7	0.7	0.9	0.92
0.5	0.5	0.5	0.9	1.80
0.5	0.9	0.9	0.9	0.56

we see, how differences in the observation rates can influence the bias ratio dramatically. In general neither the condition $q_{0j} < q_{1j}$ nor the condition $q_{i1} < q_{ij} \forall i$ are sufficient to determine, whether over- or underestimation of ϕ_j^* occurs. However, the bias ratio can be estimated, as the observation probabilities q_{ij} can be estimated. For details, see Vach & Blettner (1991). Further it should be noted, that the bias ratio is not a direct function of the overall observation rate: If we change the observation rates q_{ij} proportionally the bias ratio does not change.

The above considerations can be summarized in the following two statements. In the analysis of prospective studies we can expect to yield consistent estimates by Complete Case Analysis, as the observation probabilities do not depend on the outcome variable. In retrospective studies the estimates of a Complete Case Analysis may be biased or not; the dangerous situation is characterized by a simultaneous dependence of the observation probabilities on the outcome variable *and* a covariate.

References

Complete Case Analysis is the standard approach to handling missing values in most statistical software packages. It is often thought that the loss of efficiency in the only problem associated with its use, e.g. Miettinen (1985, p. 231) writes: "The "cleanest" way of coping with missing data is to *delete* from the analysis those subjects on whom information is missing on any of the relevant characteristics; this is the only approach that assures that no bias is introduced under any circumstances." The possible bias when used in the analysis of case-control studies was demonstrated by Vach & Blettner (1991).

4.5 Additional Category

The Method

The $(K + 1)$th category of Z_2 is just regarded as an ordinary category of the second covariate, for which an additional regression parameter β_{2K+1} is introduced. Hence the analysis is based on the modeling

$$P(Y = 1|X_1 = j, Z_2 = k) = \Lambda(\beta_0 + \beta_{1j} + \beta_{2k}) \tag{4.13}$$

Asymptotic Bias

For the cell probabilities of the contingency table $(n_{ijk})_{i=0,1;j=1,\dots,J;k=1,\dots,K+1}$ we find

$$p_{ijk}^{ADD} = P(Y = i, X_1 = j, Z_2 = k)$$

$$= \begin{cases} q_{ijk} p_{ijk}^* & \text{if } k \neq ? \\ \sum_{k'=1}^{K} (1 - q_{ijk'}) p_{ijk'}^* & \text{if } k = ? \end{cases}.$$

Hence for the odds ratios in this table we have for $k \neq ?$

$$\phi_{jk}^{ADD} = \phi_{jk}^{CC} \quad \text{and} \quad \psi_{jk}^{ADD} = \psi_{jk}^{CC}$$

and

$$\phi_{j?}^{ADD} = \frac{\left[\sum_{k'=1}^{K}(1 - q_{1jk'})p_{1jk'}^*\right]\left[\sum_{k'=1}^{K}(1 - q_{01k'})p_{01k'}^*\right]}{\left[\sum_{k'=1}^{K}(1 - q_{0jk'})p_{0jk'}^*\right]\left[\sum_{k'=1}^{K}(1 - q_{11k'})p_{11k'}^*\right]}$$

and

$$\psi_{j?}^{ADD} = \frac{\left[\sum_{k'=1}^{K}(1 - q_{1jk'})p_{1jk'}^*\right]q_{0j1}p_{0j1}^*}{\left[\sum_{k'=1}^{K}(1 - q_{0jk'})p_{0jk'}^*\right]q_{1j1}p_{1j1}^*}.$$

Hence for the odds ratios not involving the additional categories the situation is equal to Complete Case Analysis (cf. Section 4.4). If Additional Category would be a serious method then $\phi_{j?}^{ADD}$ should be related to ϕ_j^* and $\psi_{j?}^{ADD}$ should be independent of j. Instead $\phi_{j?}^{ADD}$ is related to the pooled odds ratio

$$\phi_j^{POOL} := \frac{p_{1j.}^* p_{01.}^*}{p_{0j.}^* p_{11.}^*}$$

which becomes most obvious under the MAR assumption $q_{ijk} \equiv q_{ij}$, because then

$$\phi_{j?}^{ADD} = \phi_j^{POOL} \frac{(1 - q_{1j})(1 - q_{01})}{(1 - q_{0j})(1 - q_{11})}.$$

If moreover $q_{ijk} \equiv q_i$ or $q_{ijk} \equiv q_j$ then $\phi_{j?}^{ADD} = \phi_j^{POOL}$, i.e., we have K strata with the true odds ratio and one additional stratum with the odds ratio from the pooled data, and the resulting estimate will be anywhere between these values. Hence the estimate of ϕ_j is biased, except if $\phi_j^{POOL} = \phi_j^*$, i.e. if the second covariate is no confounder. It is not surprising that in the stratum defined by the additional category the pooled odds ratio appears, because for these units X_2 is unknown.

Furthermore there are no conditions on the missing value mechanism which imply that $\psi_{j?}^{ADD}$ is independent of j.

Regarding missing values as an additional category is very similar to the imputation of unconditional probabilities considered in the next section. Comparing the modeling (4.13) with that of imputation of unconditional or conditional probabilities ((4.14) and (4.15)) we recognize that both neglect the dependence on X_1 for finding an appropriate guess for the missing value.

Summarizing, if we want to estimate the effect of X_1, but we have to adjust for a confounder X_2 for which we can observe only Z_2 affected by missing values, then Additional Category is no wise strategy to handle missing values.

References

Regarding missing values in a confounding variable as an additional category is widespread in epidemiology. The inadequacy of this approach was demonstrated by Vach & Blettner (1991).

4.6 Probability Imputation

The Method

Assuming a binary covariate X_2, the idea of Probability Imputation is to replace a missing value by an estimate for its expectation. For continuous covariates this approach is known as mean imputation (Buck 1960; Afifi & Elashoff 1966; Beale & Little 1975). As for a binary variable the expectation equals the probability to be 1, this approach can be called Probability Imputation. If X_2 has several categories, we can regard each category as a binary dummy variable and apply Probability Imputation to each dummy variable. The completed data set is then analyzed by logistic regression, regarding X_2 or the dummy variables as continuous ones.

We have to distinguish two types of Probability Imputation. The first one imputes the simple estimates

$$\hat{\pi}_k^U := \frac{n_{..k}}{n_{..+}} \,,$$

in the second the imputed value depends on the value of the first covariate X_1, i.e., we use one of the values

$$\hat{\pi}_{k|j}^n = \frac{n_{.jk}}{n_{.j+}} \,,$$

previously used in the PML Estimation (cf. Section 4.2). We refer to these two types as Unconditional Probability Imputation (UPI) and Conditional Probability Imputation (CPI).

Probability Imputation as an Approximation to PML Estimation

The completed data set is analyzed using the implicit modeling

$$P(Y = 1|X_1 = j, Z_2 = ?) = \Lambda(\beta_0 + \beta_{1j} + \sum_{k'=1}^{K} \hat{\pi}_{k'}^{U} \beta_{2k'}) \tag{4.14}$$

or

$$P(Y = 1|X_1 = j, Z_2 = ?) = \Lambda(\beta_0 + \beta_{1j} + \sum_{k'=1}^{K} \hat{\pi}_{k'|j}^{n} \beta_{2k'}) . \tag{4.15}$$

In Section 4.2 we have seen that the modeling

$$P(Y = 1|X_1 = j, Z_2 = ?) = \sum_{k'=1}^{K} \hat{\pi}_{k'|j}^{n} \Lambda(\beta_0 + \beta_{1j} + \beta_{2k'})$$

is appropriate. (For $Z_2 \neq ?$ the modeling of the three approaches coincides.) The difference between these three modelings is illustrated in Figure 4.1 for the case of a dichotomous X_2: Imputation of conditional probabilities would be an exact approximation to PML Estimation, if Λ is linear. However, Λ is not linear and the difference seems to be large in the figure, but here we assumed a value of 4 for β_{22}. If the influence of X_2 is smaller, the approximation seems to be much better. Nevertheless we have to expect that CPI results in biased estimates. However, UPI must be regarded as a much worse approximation, and hence we expect that the bias of UPI is larger than the bias of CPI. Only if X_1 and X_2 are independent, UPI seems to be as appropriate as CPI.

Even if we yield nearly unbiased estimates, it remains the problem of the underestimation of variance. In the formula of the asymptotic variance of the the PML estimate the second term represents a correction due to the estimation of π. Variance estimation based on the data set completed by Probability Imputation neglects this term. Hence we have to expect that the variance estimates are systematically to small.

The idea of an approximation of PML Estimation by Probability Imputation and our considerations in Section 4.2 about the extension to the general MAR case imply that for missing value mechanisms satisfying the MAR but not the MDX assumption we have to use the estimates $\tilde{\pi}^n$ defined by (4.6) instead of $\hat{\pi}^n$ for Conditional Probability Imputation.

References

Imputation of means for missing values is perhaps one of the oldest methods to deal with missing values in continuous covariates. An early mentioning can be found in Wilks (1932). It can be supposed that it has been also used for binary variables in many applications. Probability Imputation has been recently recommended by Schemper & Smith (1990).

In the literature one can also find the suggestion to condition not only on the covariates, but also on the outcome variable (e.g. Buck 1960). Considering Probability Imputation as an approximation to PML Estimation gives no hint to do this.

$\Lambda(x)$

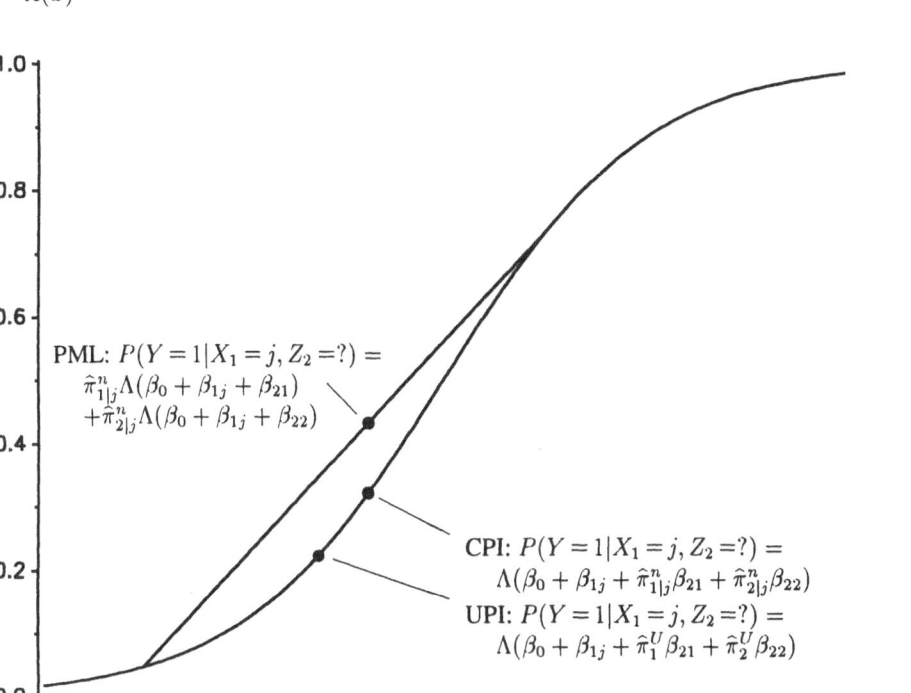

Figure 4.1: Approximation of the modeling of PML Estimation by Conditional Probability Imputation and Unconditional Probability Imputation

4.7 Omission of Covariate

The Method

The covariate X_2 is excluded from the analysis. The remaining data is analyzed according to the model

$$P(Y=1|X_1=j) = \Lambda(\beta_0 + \beta_{1j}) \ .$$

Asymptotic Bias

Omission of Covariate implies a biased estimation of β_{1j}. The asymptotic bias can be explicitly derived by comparing the wrong modeling above with the correct modeling

$$P(Y = 1|X_1 = j) = \sum_{k=1}^{K} \pi_{k|j} \Lambda(\beta_0 + \beta_{1j} + \beta_{2k}) .$$

From this comparison we can conclude that the estimate of β_0 tends to

$$\Lambda^{-1}[\sum_{k=1}^{K} \pi_{k|1} \Lambda(\beta_0^0 + \beta_{2k}^0)]$$

and that the estimate of β_{1j} tends to

$$\Lambda^{-1}[\sum_{k=1}^{K} \pi_{k|j} \Lambda(\beta_0^0 + \beta_{1j}^0 + \beta_{2k}^0)] - \Lambda^{-1}[\sum_{k=1}^{K} \pi_{k|1} \Lambda(\beta_0^0 + \beta_{2k}^0)] ;$$

hence the asymptotic bias of the estimate of β_{1j} is equal to

$$\Lambda^{-1}[\sum_{k=1}^{K} \pi_{k|j} \Lambda(\beta_0^0 + \beta_{1j}^0 + \beta_{2k}^0)] - \Lambda^{-1}[\sum_{k=1}^{K} \pi_{k|1} \Lambda(\beta_0^0 + \beta_{2k}^0)] - \beta_{1j}^0 .$$

This expression allows two important observations. First, if the covariates are independent, i.e., if $\pi_{k|1} \equiv \pi_{k|j}$, then we cannot conclude that the bias vanishes, because Λ is not linear. However, Λ may be linear enough to expect only a bias of negligible magnitude. Second, if the covariates are dependent, then even if we regard Λ as nearly linear it remains a bias of approximatively

$$\sum_{k=1}^{K} (\pi_{k|j} - \pi_{k|1}) \beta_{2k} .$$

Compared to Probability Imputation one may expect that the bias of Omission of Covariate is larger, because the first method uses a wrong modeling for units with a missing information in X_2, whereas the second uses a wrong modeling for all units.

It is worth mentioning that the estimates of the variance of the regression parameters tend to be much smaller than the corresponding estimates using the maximum likelihood principle (Section 4.1). First in a logistic model maximum likelihood estimates of an effect without adjustment for additional covariates are more precise than maximum likelihood estimates with adjustment (Robinson & Jewell 1991) and second the maximum likelihood estimates based on complete data are more precise than the maximum likelihood estimates based on incomplete data. Hence considering Omission of Covariate as a tool to handle missing value the bias of the estimation is accompanied with a tendency to smaller confidence intervals.

References

The necessity to adjust the estimation of the effect of one covariate for the effects of other covariates is widely discussed in the statistical literature. Especially in epidemiology the handling of confounding risk factors plays a fundamental role (cf. Breslow & Day 1980). An analytical treatment of the bias due to the omission of covariates is given by Gail, Wieand & Piantadosi (1984).

5. Quantitative Comparisons: Asymptotic Results

So far the evaluation of the methods has been performed on a qualitative level: We have three consistent methods (ML Estimation, PML Estimation and Filling) and four asymptotically biased methods (Conditional and Unconditional Probability Imputation, Additional Category and Omission of Covariate). The bias of Complete Case Analysis is of another quality, because it depends only on the structure of the missing rates. With the exception of MDXY mechanisms, Complete Case Analysis yields consistent estimates for the regression parameters β_{1j} and β_{2k}, and hence it can be compared to the three consistent methods mentioned above.

In this chapter we continue the evaluation on a quantitative level. We start with comparing the three consistent methods by means of asymptotic relative efficiency (Sections 5.1 to 5.3). Here the asymptotic relative efficiency between two estimates $\hat{\zeta}$ and $\hat{\hat{\zeta}}$ both consistent for a real-valued parameter ζ is defined as the ratio between their asymptotic variances; i.e.,

$$ARE(\zeta) := \frac{\lim_{n \to \infty} Var(\sqrt{n}(\hat{\zeta} - \zeta^0))}{\lim_{n \to \infty} Var(\sqrt{n}(\hat{\hat{\zeta}} - \zeta^0))} .$$

A value less than 1.0 indicates that $\hat{\zeta}$ gives more accurate estimates than $\hat{\hat{\zeta}}$ and it can be regarded as the fraction of units necessary to gain the same accuracy using $\hat{\zeta}$ instead of $\hat{\hat{\zeta}}$. As ML Estimation is efficient, PML Estimation and the Filling method can show an ARE only less or equal to 1.0.

In Section 5.4 we consider the gain of ML Estimation compared to Complete Case Analysis for those constellations, where the latter gives consistent estimates. Here we want to judge the reward for our efforts, we expect a substantial gain. However, even impressive results here may be somewhat misleading, because Complete Case Analysis is a method wasteful of information, and hence they may fake that ML Estimation solve the problem of missing values. To evaluate the loss due to missing values *only* we investigate in Section 5.5 the asymptotic relative efficiency between ML Estimation for complete data and ML Estimation for incomplete data, i.e., between the two approaches efficient for their problems. In contrast the evaluation of the asymptotic relative efficiency between ML Estimation of complete data and Complete Case Analysis of incomplete data in Section 5.6 focuses on the loss due to missing values *and* the use of an inappropriate method. A summary of the comparisons by means of asymptotic relative efficiency is given in Section 5.7.

For the four asymptotically biased methods we have given in Chapter 4 a qualitative comparison by considering the approximation to PML Estimation. A quantitative comparison can be based on the asymptotic bias, which can be easily computed by solving the equations

$$E_{\beta^0} \frac{\partial}{\partial \beta} \tilde{\ell}(\beta; Y, X_1, Z_2) = 0$$

for β where $\tilde{\ell}$ is the loglikelihood according to the implicit modeling of the methods and the estimates of $\pi_{k|j}$ are substituted by their stochastic limits. Our qualitative comparison showed that the correlation between the covariates was the crucial point for these methods with the exception of Conditional Probability Imputation. Hence in Section 5.8 we present some results about the magnitude of the asymptotic bias in dependence of the correlation. Then in Section 5.9 we consider the asymptotic bias of Conditional Probability Imputation in more detail. As pointed out in Section 4.6 bias is only one problem, the other is the underestimation of variance due to a lack of correction for the estimation of imputed probabilities. A first impression of the magnitude of this lack can be achieved by considering the portion of the variance in the PML approach, which is due to the estimation of π. This investigation is presented in Section 5.10.

The final Section 5.11 considers the asymptotic relative efficiency between ML Estimation for complete data and Filling. Because the incorrect, naive variance estimate from the filled table is an estimate for the asymptotic variance of the maximum likelihood estimate based on complete data, this investigation gives us also some information, to what degree the variance correction of the Filling method is necessary.

The main conceptual problem in this chapter is the large number of parameters on which the quantities of interest depend. We restrict our investigation to the case of two dichotomous covariates, but even then there remain the following ten parameters:

$p_1 := P(X_1 = 2),$ describing the distribution of the first covariate;

$p_2 := P(X_2 = 2),$ describing the distribution of the second covariate;

$\rho := corr(X_1, X_2),$ the correlation between the covariates;

$\beta_1 := \beta_{12}, \beta_2 := \beta_{22},$ the regression coefficients;

$\gamma := P(Y = 1),$ which is a one-to-one correspondence to the intercept β_0,

                           given $\beta_1, \beta_2, p_1, p_2, \rho$;

$q_{01}, q_{02}, q_{11}, q_{12},$ the four observation probabilities.

Even if we would succeed in presenting explicit formulas for the quantities of interest [6†], it is rather questionable whether they will be simple enough to see the desired relations. Our strategy to achieve some insights into the dependency on the parameters consists of two steps: We first consider six choices for the parameters $p_1, p_2, \rho, \gamma, q_{01}, q_{02}, q_{11}, q_{12}$ and for each of these six designs we vary the regression parameters β_1 and β_2 from -2 to 2 by a stepwidth of 1. The six designs are:

	p_1	p_2	ρ	γ	q_{01}	q_{02}	q_{11}	q_{12}
D1	0.5	0.5	0.0	0.5	0.7	0.7	0.7	0.7
D2	0.5	0.5	0.5	0.5	0.7	0.7	0.7	0.7
D3	0.2	0.2	0.0	0.2	0.7	0.7	0.7	0.7
D4	0.5	0.5	0.0	0.5	0.5	0.9	0.5	0.9
D5	0.5	0.5	0.0	0.5	0.5	0.5	0.9	0.9
D6	0.5	0.5	0.0	0.5	0.5	0.7	0.7	0.9

In the first three designs the MCAR assumption holds. The design D2 aims to evaluate the influence of correlation between the covariates, as this is the only alteration compared to D1.

[6†] For the asymptotic relative efficiencies this is possible in principle, because we have explicit formulas for the asymptotic variances of our methods. But due to the occurrence of inverses in this formulas it is cumbersome to achieve them.

The design D3 differs from D1 by an imbalance of the distribution of the covariates and of the outcome variable. The last three designs aim to evaluate the influence of the type of the missing mechanism. D4 is an example for MDX, D5 an example for MDY and D6 for MDXY missing value mechanisms. For all these designs and all choices of the regression parameters the overall observation rate is 0.7. Because of symmetry it suffices to consider nonnegative values of the regression parameters for the designs D1, D4, and D5.

In the second step we carry out *worst case analyses*. We focus here on the worst possible efficiency (or bias) given a choice for the missing rates and varying the other parameters. The values considered within this variation are all combinations of the following values for the single parameters:

$$p_1: \qquad 0.2 \text{ to } 0.8 \text{ by } 0.1$$
$$p_2: \qquad 0.2 \text{ to } 0.8 \text{ by } 0.1$$
$$\rho: \qquad -0.8 \text{ to } 0.8 \text{ by } 0.1 \ ^{7\dagger)}$$
$$\gamma: \qquad 0.2 \text{ to } 0.8 \text{ by } 0.1$$
$$\beta_1, \beta_2: \quad -2.0 \text{ to } 2.0 \text{ by } 1.0$$

Not only the worst result but also the parameter constellation where it occurs is of interest, and in general there are several such constellations. In the tables we present one of these constellations, if the other constellations can be achieved by taking $1 - p_i$ instead of p_i, $1 - \gamma$ instead of γ, or changing the sign of ρ or of the regression parameters. If a parameter can be varied over its whole range without changing the worst result, this is indicated by a dash. Sets of parameter constellations which cannot be represented this way are indicated by the word "many". For some investigations we conduct also a worst case analysis with further parameter restrictions like $\rho = 0$ or $\beta_2 = 0$.

For each worst case analysis we examine the following 8 choices for the missing rates, covering a moderate (M) and an extreme (E) choice for each of the four types of missing value mechanism MCAR, MDX, MDY, and MDXY:

	q_{01}	q_{02}	q_{11}	q_{12}
MCAR-M	0.7	0.7	0.7	0.7
MCAR-E	0.3	0.3	0.3	0.3
MDX-M	0.5	0.9	0.5	0.9
MDX-E	0.1	0.9	0.1	0.9
MDY-M	0.5	0.5	0.9	0.9
MDY-E	0.1	0.1	0.9	0.9
MDXY-M	0.5	0.7	0.7	0.9
MDXY-E	0.1	0.5	0.5	0.9

Note that, with the exception of MCAR, the overall observation rate is varying with the variation of the parameters $p_1, p_2, \rho, \gamma, \beta_1, \beta_2$, and that this variation covers approximately the whole range of the observation rates $q_{01}, q_{02}, q_{11}, q_{12}$.

[7†)] The range of ρ was restricted for some combinations of p_1 and p_2 to exclude undefined constellations and constellations with a cell probability of 0.

We have to emphasize that the results which we will present are only based on numerical computations for certain parameter constellations. Hence we are only able to formulate conjectures; analytical proofs are not given.

5.1 Asymptotic Relative Efficiency: ML Estimation vs. PML Estimation

In Section 4.2 we have introduced two estimates for the regression parameters differing in the estimates of the nuisance parameter π.. We refer to these methods as PMLX if π is estimated by $\hat{\pi}^n$ defined by (4.5) or as PMLY if π is estimated by $\tilde{\pi}^n$ defined by (4.6). PMLX should be only used under the MDX assumption.

Comparing ML Estimation and PMLX with respect to the asymptotic relative efficiency of β_1 the results for the four designs D1 to D4 in Table 5.1 indicate that we have a loss of efficiency if $\beta_2 \neq 0$, and that the loss is small in general. The result of the worst case analysis in Table 5.2 establish this: if $\beta_2 = 0$ no loss of efficiency is observed, and otherwise the loss is rather negligible for the moderate designs (ARE > 0.99) and only larger in the extreme designs. With respect to the estimation of β_2 no design with an asymptotic relative efficiency not equal to 1.0 could be found.

Comparing ML and PMLY, the results of Tables 5.3 and 5.4 indicate no loss of efficiency with respect to the estimation of β_1 for the MCAR and MDX missing value mechanisms. For the moderate MDY and MDXY choices the loss is again negligible, but may reach a substantial magnitude in the extreme designs. Neither $\beta_2 = 0$ nor $\rho = 0$ prevent a loss of efficiency, but both restrictions together do. With respect to the estimation of β_2 we have similar results (Table 5.5), except that the joint restriction $\beta_2 = 0$ and $\rho = 0$ does not imply an ARE of 1.0.

The most surprising result of this section is the uniform superiority of PMLY to PMLX. This implies that even in situations were the use of the simple estimate $\hat{\pi}^n$ is justified, it may be better from the point of asymptotic relative efficiency to use the estimate $\tilde{\pi}^n$. Moreover in these situations its use implies an efficient estimation of the regression parameters. A possible explanation may be that $\tilde{\pi}^n$ is always the maximum likelihood estimate for π under a multinomial model for the joint distribution of (Y, X_1, X_2) and the MAR assumption.

D1
$p_1=0.5$, $p_2=0.5$, $\rho=0.0$, $\gamma=0.5$
$q_{0j}\equiv0.7$

		β_1		
		0.0	1.0	2.0
β_2	0.0	1.0000	1.0000	1.0000
	1.0	0.9999	0.9999	0.9999
	2.0	0.9986	0.9988	0.9992

D2
$p_1=0.5$, $p_2=0.5$, $\rho=0.5$, $\gamma=0.5$
$q_{0j}\equiv0.7$

		β_1				
		-2.0	-1.0	0.0	1.0	2.0
β_2	-2.0	0.9991	0.9991	0.9993	0.9996	0.9998
	-1.0	0.9999	0.9999	0.9999	$0.999\bar{9}$	$0.999\bar{9}$
	0.0	1.0000	1.0000	1.0000	1.0000	1.0000
	1.0	$0.999\bar{9}$	$0.999\bar{9}$	0.9999	0.9999	0.9999
	2.0	0.9998	0.9996	0.9993	0.9991	0.9991

D3
$p_1=0.2$, $p_2=0.2$, $\rho=0.0$, $\gamma=0.2$
$q_{0j}\equiv0.7$

		β_1				
		-2.0	-1.0	0.0	1.0	2.0
β_2	-2.0	0.9999	0.9999	0.9999	0.9999	0.9997
	-1.0	$0.999\bar{9}$	$0.999\bar{9}$	$0.999\bar{9}$	$0.999\bar{9}$	0.9999
	0.0	1.0000	1.0000	1.0000	1.0000	1.0000
	1.0	$0.999\bar{9}$	$0.999\bar{9}$	$0.999\bar{9}$	0.9999	0.9999
	2.0	0.9998	0.9996	0.9993	0.9993	0.9995

D4
$p_1=0.5$, $p_2=0.5$, $\rho=0.0$, $\gamma=0.5$
$q_{i0}\equiv0.5$, $q_{i1}\equiv0.9$

		β_1		
		0.0	1.0	2.0
β_2	0.0	1.0000	1.0000	1.0000
	1.0	0.9996	0.9996	0.9997
	2.0	0.9950	0.9958	0.9974

Table 5.1: Asymptotic relative efficiency with respect to the estimation of β_1 between ML Estimation and PMLX. The entries $0.999\bar{9}$ indicate a value larger then 0.99995 but smaller then 1.0000.

observability rates				parameter restrictions						minimal $ARE(\beta_1)$	parameter constellations with minimal $ARE(\beta_1)$						
q_{01}	q_{02}	q_{11}	q_{12}	p_1	p_2	ρ	γ	β_1	β_2		p_1	p_2	ρ	γ	β_1	β_2	q^A
MCAR-M	0.7	0.7	0.7	0.7	−	−	−	−	−	−	0.99856	0.5	0.5	0.0	0.5	0.0	-2.0	0.70
MCAR-E	0.3	0.3	0.3	0.3	−	−	−	−	−	−	0.96354	0.5	0.5	0.0	0.5	0.0	-2.0	0.30
MDX-M	0.5	0.9	0.5	0.9	−	−	−	−	−	−	0.99240	0.8	0.5	0.0	0.5	0.0	-2.0	0.82
MDX-E	0.1	0.9	0.1	0.9	−	−	−	−	−	−	0.88803	0.8	0.5	0.0	0.5	0.0	-2.0	0.74
MCAR-M	0.7	0.7	0.7	0.7	−	−	−	−	−	0.0	1.00000	all						
MCAR-E	0.3	0.3	0.3	0.3	−	−	−	−	−	0.0	1.00000	all						
MDX-M	0.5	0.9	0.5	0.9	−	−	−	−	−	0.0	1.00000	all						
MDX-E	0.1	0.9	0.1	0.9	−	−	−	−	−	0.0	1.00000	all						

Table 5.2: Asymptotic relative efficiency with respect to the estimation of β_1 between ML Estimation and PMLX. Results of worst case analysis.

D1
$p_1=0.5,\ p_2=0.5,\ \rho=0.0,\ \gamma=0.5$
$q_{0j}\equiv0.7$

		β_1		
		0.0	1.0	2.0
	0.0	1.0000	1.0000	1.0000
β_2	1.0	1.0000	1.0000	1.0000
	2.0	1.0000	1.0000	1.0000

D2
$p_1=0.5,\ p_2=0.5,\ \rho=0.5,\ \gamma=0.5$
$q_{0j}\equiv0.7$

		β_1				
		-2.0	-1.0	0.0	1.0	2.0
	-2.0	1.0000	1.0000	1.0000	1.0000	1.0000
	-1.0	1.0000	1.0000	1.0000	1.0000	1.0000
β_2	0.0	1.0000	1.0000	1.0000	1.0000	1.0000
	1.0	1.0000	1.0000	1.0000	1.0000	1.0000
	2.0	1.0000	1.0000	1.0000	1.0000	1.0000

D3
$p_1=0.2,\ p_2=0.2,\ \rho=0.0,\ \gamma=0.2$
$q_{0j}\equiv0.7$

		β_1				
		-2.0	-1.0	0.0	1.0	2.0
	-2.0	1.0000	1.0000	1.0000	1.0000	1.0000
	-1.0	1.0000	1.0000	1.0000	1.0000	1.0000
β_2	0.0	1.0000	1.0000	1.0000	1.0000	1.0000
	1.0	1.0000	1.0000	1.0000	1.0000	1.0000
	2.0	1.0000	1.0000	1.0000	1.0000	1.0000

D4
$p_1=0.5,\ p_2=0.5,\ \rho=0.0,\ \gamma=0.5$
$q_{i0}\equiv0.5,\ q_{i1}\equiv0.9$

		β_1		
		0.0	1.0	2.0
	0.0	1.0000	1.0000	1.0000
β_2	1.0	1.0000	1.0000	1.0000
	2.0	1.0000	1.0000	1.0000

D5
$p_1=0.5,\ p_2=0.5,\ \rho=0.0,\ \gamma=0.5$
$q_{0j}\equiv0.5,\ q_{1j}\equiv0.9$

		β_1		
		0.0	1.0	2.0
	0.0	1.0000	1.0000	1.0000
β_2	1.0	0.9994	0.9995	0.9996
	2.0	0.9984	0.9987	0.9992

D6
$p_1=0.5,\ p_2=0.5,\ \rho=0.0,\ \gamma=0.5$
$q_{00}=0.5,\ q_{01}=0.7,\ q_{10}=0.7,\ q_{11}=0.9$

		β_1				
		-2.0	-1.0	0.0	1.0	2.0
	0.0	1.0000	1.0000	1.0000	1.0000	1.0000
β_2	1.0	0.9999	0.9998	0.9998	0.9998	0.9999
	2.0	0.9997	0.9996	0.9995	0.9996	0.9998

Table 5.3: Asymptotic relative efficiency with respect to the estimation of β_1 between ML Estimation and PMLY.

observability rates				parameter restrictions						minimal $ARE(\beta_1)$	parameter constellations with minimal $ARE(\beta_1)$						
q_{01}	q_{02}	q_{11}	q_{12}	p_1	p_2	ρ	γ	β_1	β_2		p_1	p_2	ρ	γ	β_1	β_2	q^A
MCAR-M	0.7	0.7	0.7	0.7	–	–	–	–	–	–	1.00000	all						
MCAR-E	0.3	0.3	0.3	0.3	–	–	–	–	–	–	1.00000	all						
MDX-M	0.5	0.9	0.5	0.9	–	–	–	–	–	–	1.00000	all						
MDX-E	0.1	0.9	0.1	0.9	–	–	–	–	–	–	1.00000	all						
MDY-M	0.5	0.5	0.9	0.9	–	–	–	–	–	–	0.99778	0.2	0.4	0.1	0.3	0.0	2.0	0.62
MDY-E	0.1	0.1	0.9	0.9	–	–	–	–	–	–	0.80632	–	0.5	0.0	0.3	0.0	-2.0	0.34
MDXY-M	0.5	0.7	0.7	0.9	–	–	–	–	–	–	0.99910	0.8	0.5	-0.1	0.4	0.0	-2.0	0.74
MDXY-E	0.1	0.5	0.5	0.9	–	–	–	–	–	–	0.85774	0.8	0.4	-0.2	0.4	0.0	-2.0	0.58
MDY-M	0.5	0.5	0.9	0.9	–	–	–	–	–	0.0	0.99949	0.4	0.5	-0.7	0.8	-2.0	0.0	0.82
MDY-E	0.1	0.1	0.9	0.9	–	–	–	–	–	0.0	0.94125	0.4	0.5	-0.7	0.8	-2.0	0.0	0.26
MDXY-M	0.5	0.7	0.7	0.9	–	–	–	–	–	0.0	0.99992	0.8	0.2	-0.8	0.2	-2.0	0.0	0.70
MDXY-E	0.1	0.5	0.5	0.9	–	–	–	–	–	0.0	0.93953	0.7	0.3	-0.8	0.2	-2.0	0.0	0.46
MDY-M	0.5	0.5	0.9	0.9	–	–	0.0	–	–	–	0.99779	–	0.4	0.0	0.3	0.0	2.0	0.62
MDY-E	0.1	0.1	0.9	0.9	–	–	0.0	–	–	–	0.80632	–	0.5	0.0	0.3	0.0	2.0	0.34
MDXY-M	0.5	0.7	0.7	0.9	–	–	0.0	–	–	–	0.99912	0.8	0.5	0.0	0.4	0.0	-2.0	0.80
MDXY-E	0.1	0.5	0.5	0.9	–	–	0.0	–	–	–	0.86497	0.8	0.4	0.0	0.3	-1.0	-2.0	0.54
MDY-M	0.5	0.5	0.9	0.9	–	–	0.0	–	–	0.0	1.00000	all						
MDY-E	0.1	0.1	0.9	0.9	–	–	0.0	–	–	0.0	1.00000	all						
MDXY-M	0.5	0.7	0.7	0.9	–	–	0.0	–	–	0.0	1.00000	all						
MDXY-E	0.1	0.5	0.5	0.9	–	–	0.0	–	–	0.0	1.00000	all						

Table 5.4: Asymptotic relative efficiency with respect to the estimation of β_1 between ML Estimation and PMLY. Results of worst case analysis.

observability rates				parameter restrictions						minimal $ARE(\beta_2)$	parameter constellations with minimal $ARE(\beta_2)$						
q_{01}	q_{02}	q_{11}	q_{12}	p_1	p_2	ρ	γ	β_1	β_2		p_1	p_2	ρ	γ	β_1	β_2	q^A
MCAR-M 0.7	0.7	0.7	0.7	–	–	–	–	–	–	1.00000	all						
MCAR-E 0.3	0.3	0.3	0.3	–	–	–	–	–	–	1.00000	all						
MDX-M 0.5	0.9	0.5	0.9	–	–	–	–	–	–	1.00000	all						
MDX-E 0.1	0.9	0.1	0.9	–	–	–	–	–	–	1.00000	all						
MDY-M 0.5	0.5	0.9	0.9	–	–	–	–	–	–	0.99892	0.4	0.3	0.7	0.2	-2.0	1.0	0.58
MDY-E 0.1	0.1	0.9	0.9	–	–	–	–	–	–	0.88354	0.2	0.3	0.5	0.2	2.0	-2.0	0.26
MDXY-M 0.5	0.7	0.7	0.9	–	–	–	–	–	–	0.99985	0.3	0.2	0.6	0.2	-2.0	1.0	0.60
MDXY-E 0.1	0.5	0.5	0.9	–	–	–	–	–	–	0.92554	0.3	0.2	0.5	0.2	-2.0	1.0	0.30
MDY-M 0.5	0.5	0.9	0.9	–	–	–	–	–	0.0	0.99923	0.4	0.4	-0.5	0.8	-2.0	0.0	0.82
MDY-E 0.1	0.1	0.9	0.9	–	–	–	–	–	0.0	0.91598	0.4	0.3	0.7	0.2	-2.0	0.0	0.26
MDXY-M 0.5	0.7	0.7	0.9	–	–	–	–	–	0.0	0.99988	0.4	0.2	0.4	0.7	2.0	0.0	0.72
MDXY-E 0.1	0.5	0.5	0.9	–	–	–	–	–	0.0	0.92743	0.2	0.2	0.8	0.4	-2.0	0.0	0.34
MDY-M 0.5	0.5	0.9	0.9	–	–	0.0	–	–	–	0.99926	0.2	0.2	0.0	0.8	-2.0	-1.0	0.82
MDY-E 0.1	0.1	0.9	0.9	–	–	0.0	–	–	–	0.91513	0.2	0.3	0.0	0.2	2.0	-2.0	0.34
MDXY-M 0.5	0.7	0.7	0.9	–	–	0.0	–	–	–	0.99988	0.7	–	0.0	0.8	2.0	0.0	0.80
MDXY-E 0.1	0.5	0.5	0.9	–	–	0.0	–	–	–	0.92770	0.5	–	0.0	0.3	-2.0	0.0	0.42
MDY-M 0.5	0.5	0.9	0.9	–	–	0.0	–	–	0.0	0.99929	0.3	–	0.0	0.2	2.0	0.0	0.58
MDY-E 0.1	0.1	0.9	0.9	–	–	0.0	–	–	0.0	0.92535	0.4	–	0.0	0.2	2.0	0.0	0.26
MDXY-M 0.5	0.7	0.7	0.9	–	–	0.0	–	–	0.0	0.99988	0.7	–	0.0	0.2	2.0	0.0	0.68
MDXY-E 0.1	0.5	0.5	0.9	–	–	0.0	–	–	0.0	0.92770	0.5	–	0.0	0.3	-2.0	0.0	0.42

Table 5.5: Asymptotic relative efficiency with respect to the estimation of β_2 between ML Estimation and PMLY. Results of worst case analysis.

5.2 Asymptotic Relative Efficiency: ML Estimation vs. Filling

The results for the designs satisfying the MCAR assumption in Tables 5.6 and 5.7 suggest that here Filling is as efficient as ML Estimation with respect to the estimation of β_1. For the other missing value mechanisms we observe a much smaller ARE than in the comparison of ML and PML Estimation. Even in the moderate designs we can observe values between 0.9 and 0.95. For the extreme designs the loss can become very large (ARE < 0.5). As the worst results always occur for parameter constellations with a large correlation, we also conduct a worst case analysis with the further restriction $\rho = 0$ (also Table 5.7). For the moderate designs the ARE is now always larger than 0.96, but for the extreme designs we observe still large losses. Similar the restriction to $\beta_2 = 0$ shows no substantially better results. Only if $\rho = 0$ and

D1
$p_1=0.5$, $p_2=0.5$, $\rho=0.0$, $\gamma=0.5$
$q_{0j}\equiv0.7$

		β_1		
		0.0	1.0	2.0
	0.0	1.000	1.000	1.000
β_2	1.0	1.000	1.000	1.000
	2.0	1.000	1.000	1.000

D2
$p_1=0.5$, $p_2=0.5$, $\rho=0.5$, $\gamma=0.5$
$q_{0j}\equiv0.7$

		β_1				
		-2.0	-1.0	0.0	1.0	2.0
	-2.0	1.000	1.000	1.000	1.000	1.000
	-1.0	1.000	1.000	1.000	1.000	1.000
β_2	0.0	1.000	1.000	1.000	1.000	1.000
	1.0	1.000	1.000	1.000	1.000	1.000
	2.0	1.000	1.000	1.000	1.000	1.000

D3
$p_1=0.2$, $p_2=0.2$, $\rho=0.0$, $\gamma=0.2$
$q_{0j}\equiv0.7$

		β_1				
		-2.0	-1.0	0.0	1.0	2.0
	-2.0	1.000	1.000	1.000	1.000	1.000
	-1.0	1.000	1.000	1.000	1.000	1.000
β_2	0.0	1.000	1.000	1.000	1.000	1.000
	1.0	1.000	1.000	1.000	1.000	1.000
	2.0	1.000	1.000	1.000	1.000	1.000

D4
$p_1=0.5$, $p_2=0.5$, $\rho=0.0$, $\gamma=0.5$
$q_{i0}\equiv0.5$, $q_{i1}\equiv0.9$

		β_1		
		0.0	1.0	2.0
	0.0	1.000	1.000	1.000
β_2	1.0	1.000	0.998	0.994
	2.0	1.000	0.994	0.982

D5
$p_1=0.5$, $p_2=0.5$, $\rho=0.0$, $\gamma=0.5$
$q_{0j}\equiv0.5$, $q_{1j}\equiv0.9$

		β_1		
		0.0	1.0	2.0
	0.0	1.000	1.000	1.000
β_2	1.0	0.993	0.992	0.990
	2.0	0.976	0.974	0.969

D6
$p_1=0.5$, $p_2=0.5$, $\rho=0.0$, $\gamma=0.5$
$q_{00}=0.5$, $q_{01}=0.7$, $q_{10}=0.7$, $q_{11}=0.9$

		β_1				
		-2.0	-1.0	0.0	1.0	2.0
	0.0	1.000	1.000	1.000	1.000	1.000
β_2	1.0	0.992	0.995	0.998	0.999	1.000
	2.0	0.975	0.986	0.994	0.998	1.000

Table 5.6: Asymptotic relative efficiency with respect to the estimation of β_1 between ML Estimation and Filling.

$\beta_2 = 0$, the loss vanishes.

For the estimation of β_2 the results are similar (Table 5.8): No loss under MCAR, substantial loss otherwise. Note that here even the joint restriction $\rho = 0$ and $\beta_2 = 0$ does not prevent a loss of efficiency.

The influence of the variation of the observation rates on the efficiency of Filling has been also observed by Wild (1991) for the situation of completely missing covariate information. Also the simulation results of Zhao & Lipsitz (1992) demonstrate the possible loss of efficiency.

	observability rates				parameter restrictions						minimal $ARE(\beta_1)$	parameter constellations with minimal $ARE(\beta_1)$						
	q_{01}	q_{02}	q_{11}	q_{12}	p_1	p_2	ρ	γ	β_1	β_2		p_1	p_2	ρ	γ	β_1	β_2	q^A
MCAR-M	0.7	0.7	0.7	0.7	–	–	–	–	–	–	1.00000	all						
MCAR-E	0.3	0.3	0.3	0.3	–	–	–	–	–	–	1.00000	all						
MDX-M	0.5	0.9	0.5	0.9	–	–	–	–	–	–	0.92807	0.4	0.4	0.8	0.5	-2.0	2.0	0.66
MDX-E	0.1	0.9	0.1	0.9	–	–	–	–	–	–	0.38407	0.2	0.2	0.8	0.5	-2.0	-2.0	0.26
MDY-M	0.5	0.5	0.9	0.9	–	–	–	–	–	–	0.95386	0.2	0.2	0.8	0.5	-2.0	2.0	0.70
MDY-E	0.1	0.1	0.9	0.9	–	–	–	–	–	–	0.38407	0.4	0.3	0.6	0.3	-2.0	2.0	0.34
MDXY-M	0.5	0.7	0.7	0.9	–	–	–	–	–	–	0.94089	0.5	0.5	-0.8	0.5	-2.0	2.0	0.70
MDXY-E	0.1	0.5	0.5	0.9	–	–	–	–	–	–	0.43171	0.6	0.4	-0.8	0.5	-2.0	-2.0	0.54
MDX-M	0.5	0.9	0.5	0.9	–	–	0.0	–	–	–	0.98191	0.5	0.5	0.0	0.5	-2.0	-2.0	0.70
MDX-E	0.1	0.9	0.1	0.9	–	–	0.0	–	–	–	0.72139	0.3	0.5	0.0	0.4	2.0	-2.0	0.34
MDY-M	0.5	0.5	0.9	0.9	–	–	0.0	–	–	–	0.96881	0.5	0.5	0.0	0.5	-2.0	-2.0	0.70
MDY-E	0.1	0.1	0.9	0.9	–	–	0.0	–	–	–	0.56359	0.4	0.5	0.0	0.4	2.0	-2.0	0.42
MDXY-M	0.5	0.7	0.7	0.9	–	–	0.0	–	–	–	0.97529	0.5	0.5	0.0	0.5	-2.0	-2.0	0.70
MDXY-E	0.1	0.5	0.5	0.9	–	–	0.0	–	–	–	0.43171	0.6	0.5	0.0	0.4	-2.0	-2.0	0.50
MDX-M	0.5	0.9	0.5	0.9	–	–	–	–	–	0.0	0.93881	0.8	0.2	-0.8	0.3	-2.0	0.0	0.82
MDX-E	0.1	0.9	0.1	0.9	–	–	–	–	–	0.0	0.41298	0.8	0.2	-0.8	0.3	-2.0	0.0	0.74
MDY-M	0.5	0.5	0.9	0.9	–	–	–	–	–	0.0	0.98667	0.2	0.2	0.8	0.3	2.0	0.0	0.62
MDY-E	0.1	0.1	0.9	0.9	–	–	–	–	–	0.0	0.84395	0.2	0.2	0.8	0.3	2.0	0.0	0.26
MDXY-M	0.5	0.7	0.7	0.9	–	–	–	–	–	0.0	0.96620	0.2	0.2	0.8	0.7	-2.0	0.0	0.68
MDXY-E	0.1	0.5	0.5	0.9	–	–	–	–	–	0.0	0.55305	0.3	0.3	0.8	0.6	-2.0	0.0	0.46
MDX-M	0.5	0.9	0.5	0.9	–	–	0.0	–	–	0.0	1.00000	all						
MDX-E	0.1	0.9	0.1	0.9	–	–	0.0	–	–	0.0	1.00000	all						
MDY-M	0.5	0.5	0.9	0.9	–	–	0.0	–	–	0.0	1.00000	all						
MDY-E	0.1	0.1	0.9	0.9	–	–	0.0	–	–	0.0	1.00000	all						
MDXY-M	0.5	0.7	0.7	0.9	–	–	0.0	–	–	0.0	1.00000	all						
MDXY-E	0.1	0.5	0.5	0.9	–	–	0.0	–	–	0.0	1.00000	all						

Table 5.7: Asymptotic relative efficiency with respect to the estimation of β_1 between ML Estimation and Filling. Results of worst case analysis.

observability rates				parameter restrictions						minimal $ARE(\beta_2)$	parameter constellations with minimal $ARE(\beta_2)$						
q_{01}	q_{02}	q_{11}	q_{12}	p_1	p_2	ρ	γ	β_1	β_2		p_1	p_2	ρ	γ	β_1	β_2	q^A
MCAR-M	0.7	0.7	0.7	0.7	–	–	–	–	–	–	1.00000	all						
MCAR-E	0.3	0.3	0.3	0.3	–	–	–	–	–	–	1.00000	all						
MDX-M	0.5	0.9	0.5	0.9	–	–	–	–	–	–	0.91387	many						
MDX-E	0.1	0.9	0.1	0.9	–	–	–	–	–	–	0.36000	many						
MDY-M	0.5	0.5	0.9	0.9	–	–	–	–	–	–	0.95637	0.2	0.2	0.8	0.5	2.0	-2.0	0.70
MDY-E	0.1	0.1	0.9	0.9	–	–	–	–	–	–	0.60051	0.3	0.4	0.7	0.2	2.0	-2.0	0.26
MDXY-M	0.5	0.7	0.7	0.9	–	–	–	–	–	–	0.93770	0.4	0.4	-0.8	0.5	-2.0	2.0	0.68
MDXY-E	0.1	0.5	0.5	0.9	–	–	–	–	–	–	0.42668	0.3	0.3	0.8	0.5	-2.0	2.0	0.42
MDX-M	0.5	0.9	0.5	0.9	–	–	0.0	–	–	–	0.91837	many						
MDX-E	0.1	0.9	0.1	0.9	–	–	0.0	–	–	–	0.36000	many						
MDY-M	0.5	0.5	0.9	0.9	–	–	0.0	–	–	–	0.97608	0.4	0.5	0.0	0.4	2.0	-2.0	0.66
MDY-E	0.1	0.1	0.9	0.9	–	–	0.0	–	–	–	0.75911	0.3	0.5	0.0	0.3	2.0	-2.0	0.34
MDXY-M	0.5	0.7	0.7	0.9	–	–	0.0	–	–	–	0.94995	0.5	0.5	0.0	0.5	-2.0	2.0	0.70
MDXY-E	0.1	0.5	0.5	0.9	–	–	0.0	–	–	–	0.47675	0.4	0.5	0.0	0.6	-2.0	-2.0	0.50
MDX-M	0.5	0.9	0.5	0.9	–	–	–	–	–	0.0	0.91837	many						
MDX-E	0.1	0.9	0.1	0.9	–	–	–	–	–	0.0	0.36000	many						
MDY-M	0.5	0.5	0.9	0.9	–	–	–	–	–	0.0	0.98198	0.4	0.3	0.1	0.4	2.0	0.0	0.66
MDY-E	0.1	0.1	0.9	0.9	–	–	–	–	–	0.0	0.80767	0.5	0.3	-0.4	0.3	2.0	0.0	0.34
MDXY-M	0.5	0.7	0.7	0.9	–	–	–	–	–	0.0	0.95426	0.6	0.2	-0.2	0.5	-2.0	0.0	0.72
MDXY-E	0.1	0.5	0.5	0.9	–	–	–	–	–	0.0	0.49579	0.3	0.3	0.2	0.7	-2.0	0.0	0.50
MDX-M	0.5	0.9	0.5	0.9	–	–	0.0	–	–	0.0	0.91837	0.5	0.2	0.0	0.2	0.0	0.0	0.70
MDX-E	0.1	0.9	0.1	0.9	–	–	0.0	–	–	0.0	0.36000	0.0	0.2	0.0	0.2	0.0	0.0	0.70
MDY-M	0.5	0.5	0.9	0.9	–	–	0.0	–	–	0.0	0.98208	0.4	0.2	0.0	0.4	2.0	0.0	0.66
MDY-E	0.1	0.1	0.9	0.9	–	–	0.0	–	–	0.0	0.80997	0.3	0.2	0.0	0.2	2.0	0.0	0.26
MDXY-M	0.5	0.7	0.7	0.9	–	–	0.0	–	–	0.0	0.95439	0.5	0.2	0.0	0.5	-2.0	0.0	0.70
MDXY-E	0.1	0.5	0.5	0.9	–	–	0.0	–	–	0.0	0.49767	0.4	0.2	0.0	0.6	-2.0	0.0	0.50

Table 5.8: Asymptotic relative efficiency with respect to the estimation of β_2 between ML Estimation and Filling. Results of worst case analysis.

5.3 Asymptotic Relative Efficiency: PML Estimation vs. Filling

The results for the Filling method may suggest that PML Estimation is uniformly better than the Filling method. This is, with respect to the estimation of β_1, not true. For the PMLX method we have already seen that for the MCAR designs it is not efficient, whereas the Filling method shows an ARE of 1.0; hence PMLX is here worse than the Filling method. Of course, this must be true also for some MDX mechanisms being not far away from MCAR. But also for the extreme as well as for the moderate MDX design in a worst case analysis we observe parameter constellations, where PMLX is worse than the Filling method (Table 5.9).

For PMLY it is clear from the results of Section 5.1 that we cannot find a constellation where Filling is worse than PMLY in the MCAR and MDX designs. For the four other designs of missing mechanisms we always find such a constellation (Table 5.10). Hence with respect to the estimation of β_1 PMLY is not uniformly better than the Filling method.

Considering the estimation of β_2, we could not find a constellation, where PMLX or PMLY is worse than the Filling method.

	observability rates				parameter restrictions						minimal $ARE(\beta_1)$	parameter constellations with minimal $ARE(\beta_1)$						
	q_{01}	q_{02}	q_{11}	q_{12}	p_1	p_2	ρ	γ	β_1	β_2		p_1	p_2	ρ	γ	β_1	β_2	q^A
MDX-M	0.5	0.9	0.5	0.9	–	–	–	–	–	–	0.99240	0.8	0.5	0.0	0.5	0.0	-2.0	0.82
MDX-E	0.1	0.9	0.1	0.9	–	–	–	–	–	–	0.88803	0.8	0.5	0.0	0.5	0.0	-2.0	0.74

Table 5.9: Asymptotic relative efficiency with respect to the estimation of β_1 between Filling and PMLX. Results of worst case analysis.

	observability rates				parameter restrictions						minimal $ARE(\beta_2)$	parameter constellations with minimal $ARE(\beta_2)$						
	q_{01}	q_{02}	q_{11}	q_{12}	p_1	p_2	ρ	γ	β_1	β_2		p_1	p_2	ρ	γ	β_1	β_2	q^A
MDY-M	0.5	0.5	0.9	0.9	–	–	–	–	–	–	0.99959	0.2	0.3	0.6	0.8	-2.0	-1.0	0.82
MDY-E	0.1	0.1	0.9	0.9	–	–	–	–	–	–	0.94001	0.3	0.2	0.7	0.8	2.0	0.0	0.74
MDXY-M	0.5	0.7	0.7	0.9	–	–	–	–	–	–	0.99956	0.8	0.2	-0.5	0.2	-1.0	2.0	0.70
MDXY-E	0.1	0.5	0.5	0.9	–	–	–	–	–	–	0.96722	0.8	0.2	-0.6	0.2	-2.0	2.0	0.50

Table 5.10: Asymptotic relative efficiency with respect to the estimation of β_1 between Filling and PMLY. Results of worst case analysis.

5.4 Asymptotic Relative Efficiency: ML Estimation vs. Complete Case Analysis

The results of Table 5.11 demonstrate that ML Estimation can be a substantial improvement compared to Complete Case Analysis with respect to the estimation of β_1. For the MCAR mechanisms it is obvious that the loss of efficiency of Complete Case Analysis compared to an analysis of complete data without missing values is equal to the missing rate; hence the results of the designs D1 to D3 suggest that ML Estimation can overcome this loss, if $\beta_2 = 0$ and $\rho = 0$. In the next section we will show that this conjecture can be maintained also for the other missing value mechanisms, where the magnitude of the loss of Complete Case Analysis is not obvious.

From the results of the worst case analysis in Table 5.12 we can see that the ARE may be a small as the smallest missing rate, and that the parameter constellations with the largest gain are not accompanied by a small overall observation probability.

On the other hand, the values of the *maximal* ARE in Table 5.13 show that the gain can be rather small (ARE > 0.9), even if $\beta_2 = 0$. Independence of the covariates seems to prevent a small magnitude of the gain; note that here for MCAR designs the largest lost occurs for a parameter constellation, where both the covariates and the outcome variable are balanced. However, interpretation of these values is somewhat difficult, because the possible gain of ML Estimation is limited by the loss of Complete Case Analysis compared to the analysis of complete data, cf. Section 5.6.

With respect to the estimation of β_2 our computations yield always 1.0 for the ARE between ML Estimation and Complete Case Analysis.

5.5 Asymptotic Relative Efficiency: ML Estimation for Complete Data vs. ML Estimation for Incomplete Data

The ARE between ML Estimation for complete data and ML Estimation for incomplete data can be regarded as a measure for the loss caused by missing values. One may suppose that there is no loss with respect to the estimation of β_1 if $\beta_2 = 0$, because then the distribution of the outcome variable does not depend on the value of the second covariate and hence a missing value in this covariate does not matter. The results of the design D2 in Table 5.14 demonstrate that this conjecture is not true in general; however, the other five designs with uncorrelated covariates support the conjecture. Indeed, the results of the worst case analysis in Table 5.15 indicate that $\beta_2 = 0$ and $\rho = 0$ together imply an ARE of 1.0, whereas each single restriction does not. We further observe that the ARE can be much smaller than the global observation rate in the designs with varying observation rates, even if $\beta_2 = 0$. In general the parameter constellations with smallest ARE do not show a small overall observation rate. Independence of the covariates may imply a limitation of the loss of efficiency to moderate values.

With respect to the estimation of β_2 we have to expect a loss always. As the ARE of the estimation of β_2 between ML Estimation and Complete Case Analysis is equal to 1.0, the loss is equal to the loss between ML Estimation for complete data and Complete Case Analysis, which is considered in the next section.

D1
$p_1=0.5,\ p_2=0.5,\ \rho=0.0,\ \gamma=0.5$
$q_{0j}\equiv0.7$

		β_1		
		0.0	1.0	2.0
β_2	0.0	0.700	0.700	0.700
	1.0	0.718	0.721	0.728
	2.0	0.764	0.772	0.792

D2
$p_1=0.5,\ p_2=0.5,\ \rho=0.5,\ \gamma=0.5$
$q_{0j}\equiv0.7$

		β_1				
		-2.0	-1.0	0.0	1.0	2.0
β_2	-2.0	0.752	0.777	0.813	0.852	0.885
	-1.0	0.740	0.761	0.785	0.811	0.833
	0.0	0.775	0.775	0.775	0.775	0.775
	1.0	0.833	0.811	0.785	0.761	0.740
	2.0	0.885	0.852	0.813	0.777	0.752

D3
$p_1=0.2,\ p_2=0.2,\ \rho=0.0,\ \gamma=0.2$
$q_{0j}\equiv0.7$

		β_1				
		-2.0	-1.0	0.0	1.0	2.0
β_2	-2.0	0.703	0.707	0.712	0.719	0.730
	-1.0	0.701	0.703	0.705	0.708	0.712
	0.0	0.700	0.700	0.700	0.700	0.700
	1.0	0.704	0.707	0.710	0.713	0.718
	2.0	0.724	0.737	0.745	0.752	0.764

D4
$p_1=0.5,\ p_2=0.5,\ \rho=0.0,\ \gamma=0.5$
$q_{i0}\equiv0.5,\ q_{i1}\equiv0.9$

		β_1		
		0.0	1.0	2.0
β_2	0.0	0.643	0.643	0.643
	1.0	0.664	0.667	0.675
	2.0	0.719	0.728	0.750

D5
$p_1=0.5,\ p_2=0.5,\ \rho=0.0,\ \gamma=0.5$
$q_{0j}\equiv0.5,\ q_{1j}\equiv0.9$

		β_1		
		0.0	1.0	2.0
β_2	0.0	0.643	0.643	0.643
	1.0	0.663	0.666	0.674
	2.0	0.714	0.724	0.747

Table 5.11: Asymptotic relative efficiency with respect to the estimation of β_1 between ML Estimation and Complete Case Analysis.

observability rates				parameter restrictions						minimal $ARE(\beta_1)$	parameter constellations with minimal $ARE(\beta_1)$						
q_{01}	q_{02}	q_{11}	q_{12}	p_1	p_2	ρ	γ	β_1	β_2		p_1	p_2	ρ	γ	β_1	β_2	q^A
MCAR-M	0.7	0.7	0.7	0.7	–	–	–	–	–	–	0.7	many						
MCAR-E	0.3	0.3	0.3	0.3	–	–	–	–	–	–	0.3	many						
MDX-M	0.5	0.9	0.5	0.9	–	–	–	–	–	–	0.51162	0.8	–	0.0	0.2	2.0	0.0	0.82
MDX-E	0.1	0.9	0.1	0.9	–	–	–	–	–	–	0.10476	0.8	–	0.0	0.2	-2.0	0.0	0.74
MDY-M	0.5	0.5	0.9	0.9	–	–	–	–	–	–	0.51162	0.2	–	0.0	0.8	2.0	0.0	0.82
MDY-E	0.1	0.1	0.9	0.9	–	–	–	–	–	–	0.10476	0.2	–	0.0	0.8	-2.0	0.0	0.74

Table 5.12: Asymptotic relative efficiency with respect to the estimation of β_1 between ML Estimation and Filling. Results of worst case analysis.

observability rates				parameter restrictions						maximal $ARE(\beta_1)$	parameter constellations with minimal $ARE(\beta_1)$						
q_{01}	q_{02}	q_{11}	q_{12}	p_1	p_2	ρ	γ	β_1	β_2		p_1	p_2	ρ	γ	β_1	β_2	q^A
MCAR-M	0.7	0.7	0.7	0.7	–	–	–	–	–	–	0.95157	0.5	0.5	-0.8	0.5	-2.0	-2.0	0.70
MCAR-E	0.3	0.3	0.3	0.3	–	–	–	–	–	–	0.88699	0.5	0.5	-0.8	0.5	-2.0	-2.0	0.30
MDX-M	0.5	0.9	0.5	0.9	–	–	–	–	–	–	0.96772	0.2	0.2	0.8	0.4	-2.0	2.0	0.58
MDX-E	0.1	0.9	0.1	0.9	–	–	–	–	–	–	0.89907	0.2	0.3	0.7	0.2	-2.0	-2.0	0.26
MDY-M	0.5	0.5	0.9	0.9	–	–	–	–	–	–	0.95814	0.3	0.2	0.7	0.2	-2.0	2.0	0.58
MDY-E	0.1	0.1	0.9	0.9	–	–	–	–	–	–	0.88013	0.2	0.2	0.8	0.2	-2.0	2.0	0.26
MCAR-M	0.7	0.7	0.7	0.7	–	–	0.0	–	–	–	0.79245	0.5	0.5	0.0	0.5	-2.0	-2.0	0.70
MCAR-E	0.3	0.3	0.3	0.3	–	–	0.0	–	–	–	0.51571	0.5	0.5	0.0	0.5	-2.0	-2.0	0.30
MDX-M	0.5	0.9	0.5	0.9	–	–	0.0	–	–	–	0.87162	0.2	0.2	0.0	0.2	-2.0	2.0	0.58
MDX-E	0.1	0.9	0.1	0.9	–	–	0.0	–	–	–	0.66545	0.2	0.2	0.0	0.2	-2.0	2.0	0.26
MDY-M	0.5	0.5	0.9	0.9	–	–	0.0	–	–	–	0.87515	0.2	0.2	0.0	0.2	-2.0	2.0	0.58
MDY-E	0.1	0.1	0.9	0.9	–	–	0.0	–	–	–	0.69300	0.2	0.3	0.0	0.2	-2.0	2.0	0.26
MCAR-M	0.7	0.7	0.7	0.7	–	–	–	–	–	0.0	0.90064	0.2	0.2	0.8	0.2	2.0	0.0	0.70
MCAR-E	0.3	0.3	0.3	0.3	–	–	–	–	–	0.0	0.76815	0.2	0.2	0.8	0.2	2.0	0.0	0.30
MDX-M	0.5	0.9	0.5	0.9	–	–	–	–	–	0.0	0.93717	0.2	0.2	0.8	0.4	-2.0	0.0	0.58
MDX-E	0.1	0.9	0.1	0.9	–	–	–	–	–	0.0	0.88033	0.2	0.2	0.8	0.2	-2.0	0.0	0.26
MDY-M	0.5	0.5	0.9	0.9	–	–	–	–	–	0.0	0.92640	0.2	0.2	0.8	0.2	-1.0	0.0	0.58
MDY-E	0.1	0.1	0.9	0.9	–	–	–	–	–	0.0	0.83930	0.2	0.2	0.8	0.2	-2.0	0.0	0.26

Table 5.13: Asymptotic relative efficiency with respect to the estimation of β_1 between ML Estimation and Complete Case Analysis. Results of worst case analysis.

D1
$p_1=0.5$, $p_2=0.5$, $\rho=0.0$, $\gamma=0.5$
$q_{0j}\equiv0.7$

		β_1		
		0.0	1.0	2.0
	0.0	1.000	1.000	1.000
β_2	1.0	0.975	0.971	0.961
	2.0	0.916	0.906	0.883

D2
$p_1=0.5$, $p_2=0.5$, $\rho=0.5$, $\gamma=0.5$
$q_{0j}\equiv0.7$

		β_1				
		-2.0	-1.0	0.0	1.0	2.0
	-2.0	0.931	0.901	0.861	0.821	0.791
	-1.0	0.946	0.920	0.891	0.864	0.841
β_2	0.0	0.903	0.903	0.903	0.903	0.903
	1.0	0.841	0.864	0.891	0.920	0.946
	2.0	0.791	0.821	0.861	0.901	0.931

D3
$p_1=0.2$, $p_2=0.2$, $\rho=0.0$, $\gamma=0.2$
$q_{0j}\equiv0.7$

		β_1				
		-2.0	-1.0	0.0	1.0	2.0
	-2.0	0.996	0.991	0.983	0.973	0.959
	-1.0	0.998	0.996	0.993	0.989	0.983
β_2	0.0	1.000	1.000	1.000	1.000	1.000
	1.0	0.994	0.989	0.986	0.982	0.975
	2.0	0.966	0.950	0.940	0.931	0.916

D4
$p_1=0.5$, $p_2=0.5$, $\rho=0.0$, $\gamma=0.5$
$q_{i0}\equiv0.5$, $q_{i1}\equiv0.9$

		β_1		
		0.0	1.0	2.0
	0.0	1.000	1.000	1.000
β_2	1.0	0.968	0.964	0.956
	2.0	0.894	0.887	0.870

D5
$p_1=0.5$, $p_2=0.5$, $\rho=0.0$, $\gamma=0.5$
$q_{0j}\equiv0.5$, $q_{1j}\equiv0.9$

		β_1		
		0.0	1.0	2.0
	0.0	1.000	1.000	1.000
β_2	1.0	0.975	0.971	0.960
	2.0	0.916	0.906	0.881

D6
$p_1=0.5$, $p_2=0.5$, $\rho=0.0$, $\gamma=0.5$
$q_{00}=0.5$, $q_{01}=0.7$, $q_{10}=0.7$, $q_{11}=0.9$

		β_1				
		-2.0	-1.0	0.0	1.0	2.0
	0.0	1.000	1.000	1.000	1.000	1.000
β_2	1.0	0.958	0.969	0.973	0.970	0.961
	2.0	0.877	0.900	0.911	0.903	0.882

Table 5.14: Asymptotic relative efficiency with respect to the estimation of β_1 between ML Estimation for complete data and ML Estimation for incomplete data.

observability rates				parameter restrictions						minimal $ARE(\beta_1)$	parameter constellations with minimal $ARE(\beta_1)$						
q_{01}	q_{02}	q_{11}	q_{12}	p_1	p_2	ρ	γ	β_1	β_2		p_1	p_2	ρ	γ	β_1	β_2	q^A
MCAR-M	0.7	0.7	0.7	0.7	–	–	–	–	–	–	0.73563	0.5	0.5	-0.8	0.5	-2.0	-2.0	0.70
MCAR-E	0.3	0.3	0.3	0.3	–	–	–	–	–	–	0.33822	0.5	0.5	-0.8	0.5	-2.0	-2.0	0.30
MDX-M	0.5	0.9	0.5	0.9	–	–	–	–	–	–	0.61071	0.7	0.2	-0.7	0.5	-2.0	-2.0	0.78
MDX-E	0.1	0.9	0.1	0.9	–	–	–	–	–	–	0.19513	0.7	0.2	-0.7	0.4	-2.0	2.0	0.66
MDY-M	0.5	0.5	0.9	0.9	–	–	–	–	–	–	0.61788	0.3	0.2	0.7	0.6	2.0	-2.0	0.74
MDY-E	0.1	0.1	0.9	0.9	–	–	–	–	–	–	0.18156	0.2	0.2	0.7	0.5	2.0	-2.0	0.50
MDXY-M	0.5	0.7	0.7	0.9	–	–	–	–	–	–	0.61684	0.7	0.2	-0.7	0.5	-2.0	-2.0	0.74
MDXY-E	0.1	0.5	0.5	0.9	–	–	–	–	–	–	0.19756	0.7	0.2	-0.7	0.4	-2.0	-2.0	0.54
MCAR-M	0.7	0.7	0.7	0.7	–	–	–	–	–	0.0	0.77723	0.2	0.2	0.8	0.2	2.0	0.0	0.70
MCAR-E	0.3	0.3	0.3	0.3	–	–	–	–	–	0.0	0.39055	0.2	0.2	0.8	0.2	2.0	0.0	0.30
MDX-M	0.5	0.9	0.5	0.9	–	–	–	–	–	0.0	0.69448	0.2	0.3	0.7	0.2	1.0	0.0	0.58
MDX-E	0.1	0.9	0.1	0.9	–	–	–	–	–	0.0	0.29284	0.7	0.2	-0.7	0.2	-2.0	0.0	0.66
MDY-M	0.5	0.5	0.9	0.9	–	–	–	–	–	0.0	0.65521	–	0.5	0.8	0.8	0.0	0.0	0.82
MDY-E	0.1	0.1	0.9	0.9	–	–	–	–	–	0.0	0.22299	0.5	0.5	0.8	0.6	0.0	0.0	0.58
MDXY-M	0.5	0.7	0.7	0.9	–	–	–	–	–	0.0	0.68991	0.2	0.3	0.7	0.8	-2.0	0.0	0.70
MDXY-E	0.1	0.5	0.5	0.9	–	–	–	–	–	0.0	0.30552	0.2	0.3	0.7	0.7	0.0	0.0	0.46
MCAR-M	0.7	0.7	0.7	0.7	–	–	0.0	–	–	–	0.88334	0.5	0.5	0.0	0.5	-2.0	-2.0	0.70
MCAR-E	0.3	0.3	0.3	0.3	–	–	0.0	–	–	–	0.58172	0.5	0.5	0.0	0.5	-2.0	-2.0	0.30
MDX-M	0.5	0.9	0.5	0.9	–	–	0.0	–	–	–	0.84835	0.8	0.4	0.0	0.3	-2.0	-2.0	0.82
MDX-E	0.1	0.9	0.1	0.9	–	–	0.0	–	–	–	0.39344	0.8	0.5	0.0	0.5	0.0	2.0	0.74
MDY-M	0.5	0.5	0.9	0.9	–	–	0.0	–	–	–	0.85561	0.4	0.4	0.0	0.5	-2.0	-2.0	0.70
MDY-E	0.1	0.1	0.9	0.9	–	–	0.0	–	–	–	0.59294	0.4	0.4	0.0	0.4	-2.0	-2.0	0.42
MDXY-M	0.5	0.7	0.7	0.9	–	–	0.0	–	–	–	0.85783	0.6	0.4	0.0	0.4	-2.0	-2.0	0.70
MDXY-E	0.1	0.5	0.5	0.9	–	–	0.0	–	–	–	0.58449	0.6	0.4	0.0	0.3	-2.0	-2.0	0.46
MCAR-M	0.7	0.7	0.7	0.7	–	–	0.0	–	–	0.0	1.0000	all						
MCAR-E	0.3	0.3	0.3	0.3	–	–	0.0	–	–	0.0	1.0000	all						
MDX-M	0.5	0.9	0.5	0.9	–	–	0.0	–	–	0.0	1.0000	all						
MDX-E	0.1	0.9	0.1	0.9	–	–	0.0	–	–	0.0	1.0000	all						
MDY-M	0.5	0.5	0.9	0.9	–	–	0.0	–	–	0.0	1.0000	all						
MDY-E	0.1	0.1	0.9	0.9	–	–	0.0	–	–	0.0	1.0000	all						
MDXY-M	0.5	0.7	0.7	0.9	–	–	0.0	–	–	0.0	1.0000	all						
MDXY-E	0.1	0.5	0.5	0.9	–	–	0.0	–	–	0.0	1.0000	all						

Table 5.15: Asymptotic relative efficiency with respect to the estimation of β_1 between ML Estimation for complete data and ML Estimation for incomplete data. Results of worst case analysis.

5.6 Asymptotic Relative Efficiency: ML Estimation for Complete Data vs. Complete Case Analysis

The ARE between ML Estimation for complete data and Complete Case Analysis can be regarded as a measure for the loss due to the occurrence of missing values *and* the use of Complete Case Analysis. For missing value mechanisms satisfying the MCAR assumption it can be easily shown that the ARE for all regression parameters is equal to the global observation rate q^A. From the results of the designs D4 and D5 in Table 5.16 we can conclude that for MDX or MDY missing value mechanisms the ARE may be smaller than the global observation rate.

D1
$p_1=0.5$, $p_2=0.5$, $\rho=0.0$, $\gamma=0.5$
$q_{0j}\equiv0.7$

		β_1		
		0.0	1.0	2.0
	0.0	0.700	0.700	0.700
β_2	1.0	0.700	0.700	0.700
	2.0	0.700	0.700	0.700

D2
$p_1=0.5$, $p_2=0.5$, $\rho=0.5$, $\gamma=0.5$
$q_{0j}\equiv0.7$

		β_1				
		-2.0	-1.0	0.0	1.0	2.0
	-2.0	0.700	0.700	0.700	0.700	0.700
	-1.0	0.700	0.700	0.700	0.700	0.700
β_2	0.0	0.700	0.700	0.700	0.700	0.700
	1.0	0.700	0.700	0.700	0.700	0.700
	2.0	0.700	0.700	0.700	0.700	0.700

D3
$p_1=0.2$, $p_2=0.2$, $\rho=0.0$, $\gamma=0.2$
$q_{0j}\equiv0.7$

		β_1				
		-2.0	-1.0	0.0	1.0	2.0
	-2.0	0.700	0.700	0.700	0.700	0.700
	-1.0	0.700	0.700	0.700	0.700	0.700
β_2	0.0	0.700	0.700	0.700	0.700	0.700
	1.0	0.700	0.700	0.700	0.700	0.700
	2.0	0.700	0.700	0.700	0.700	0.700

D4
$p_1=0.5$, $p_2=0.5$, $\rho=0.0$, $\gamma=0.5$
$q_{i0}\equiv0.5$, $q_{i1}\equiv0.9$

		β_1		
		0.0	1.0	2.0
	0.0	0.643	0.643	0.643
β_2	1.0	0.643	0.644	0.645
	2.0	0.643	0.645	0.652

D5
$p_1=0.5$, $p_2=0.5$, $\rho=0.0$, $\gamma=0.5$
$q_{0j}\equiv0.5$, $q_{1j}\equiv0.9$

		β_1		
		0.0	1.0	2.0
	0.0	0.643	0.643	0.643
β_2	1.0	0.646	0.646	0.647
	2.0	0.654	0.655	0.658

Table 5.16: Asymptotic relative efficiency with respect to the estimation of β_1 between ML Estimation for complete data and Complete Case Analysis.

The results of the worst case analysis in Table 5.17 and 5.18 suggest that the ARE can be as small as the smallest observation rate. On the other side, looking at the *maximal* possible ARE (Table 5.19 and 5.20) we observe that there are constellations where the loss is rather small (ARE > 0.85). Moreover the parameter constellations with a small loss are neither accompanied by extreme missing rates nor extreme correlations.

observability rates				parameter restrictions						minimal $ARE(\beta_1)$	parameter constellations with minimal $ARE(\beta_1)$						
q_{01}	q_{02}	q_{11}	q_{12}	p_1	p_2	ρ	γ	β_1	β_2		p_1	p_2	ρ	γ	β_1	β_2	q^A
MCAR-M	0.7	0.7	0.7	0.7	–	–	–	–	–	–	0.7	all						
MCAR-E	0.3	0.3	0.3	0.3	–	–	–	–	–	–	0.3	all						
MDX-M	0.5	0.9	0.5	0.9	–	–	–	–	–	–	0.50919	0.8	0.4	-0.3	0.2	2.0	-2.0	0.82
MDX-E	0.1	0.9	0.1	0.9	–	–	–	–	–	–	0.10376	0.8	0.4	-0.3	0.2	-2.0	-2.0	0.58
MDY-M	0.5	0.5	0.9	0.9	–	–	–	–	–	–	0.50626	0.2	0.3	0.7	0.8	2.0	2.0	0.82
MDY-E	0.1	0.1	0.9	0.9	–	–	–	–	–	–	0.10255	0.2	0.3	0.7	0.8	2.0	2.0	0.74

Table 5.17: Asymptotic relative efficiency with respect to the estimation of β_1 between ML Estimation for complete data and Complete Case Analysis.

observability rates				parameter restrictions						minimal $ARE(\beta_2)$	parameter constellations with minimal $ARE(\beta_2)$						
q_{01}	q_{02}	q_{11}	q_{12}	p_1	p_2	ρ	γ	β_1	β_2		p_1	p_2	ρ	γ	β_1	β_2	q^A
MCAR-M	0.7	0.7	0.7	0.7	–	–	–	–	–	–	0.7	all						
MCAR-E	0.3	0.3	0.3	0.3	–	–	–	–	–	–	0.3	all						
MDX-M	0.5	0.9	0.5	0.9	–	–	–	–	–	–	0.50118	0.2	0.3	-0.3	0.2	-2.0	-2.0	0.58
MDX-E	0.1	0.9	0.1	0.9	–	–	–	–	–	–	0.10236	0.2	0.3	-0.3	0.2	-2.0	-2.0	0.26
MDY-M	0.5	0.5	0.9	0.9	–	–	–	–	–	–	0.50626	0.3	0.2	0.7	0.8	2.0	2.0	0.82
MDY-E	0.1	0.1	0.9	0.9	–	–	–	–	–	–	0.10255	0.3	0.2	0.7	0.8	2.0	2.0	0.74

Table 5.18: Asymptotic relative efficiency with respect to the estimation of β_2 between ML Estimation for complete data and Complete Case Analysis.

observability rates				parameter restrictions						maximal $ARE(\beta_1)$	parameter constellations with minimal $ARE(\beta_1)$						
q_{01}	q_{02}	q_{11}	q_{12}	p_1	p_2	ρ	γ	β_1	β_2		p_1	p_2	ρ	γ	β_1	β_2	q^A
MDX-M 0.5	0.9	0.5	0.9	–	–	–	–	–	–	0.87199	0.2	0.4	0.3	0.2	-2.0	-2.0	0.58
MDX-E 0.1	0.9	0.1	0.9	–	–	–	–	–	–	0.69348	0.2	0.3	0.4	0.2	-2.0	-2.0	0.26
MDY-M 0.5	0.5	0.9	0.9	–	–	–	–	–	–	0.88064	0.2	0.3	0.7	0.2	-2.0	-2.0	0.58
MDY-E 0.1	0.1	0.9	0.9	–	–	–	–	–	–	0.74507	0.2	0.3	0.7	0.2	-2.0	-2.0	0.26

Table 5.19: Asymptotic relative efficiency with respect to the estimation of β_1 between ML Estimation for complete data and Complete Case Analysis.

observability rates				parameter restrictions						maximal $ARE(\beta_2)$	parameter constellations with minimal $ARE(\beta_2)$						
q_{01}	q_{02}	q_{11}	q_{12}	p_1	p_2	ρ	γ	β_1	β_2		p_1	p_2	ρ	γ	β_1	β_2	q^A
MDX-M 0.5	0.9	0.5	0.9	–	–	–	–	–	–	0.89882	0.8	0.3	0.3	0.2	2.0	2.0	0.82
MDX-E 0.1	0.9	0.1	0.9							0.80764	0.8	0.3	0.3	0.2	2.0	2.0	0.74
MDY-M 0.5	0.5	0.9	0.9	–	–	–	–	–	–	0.88064	0.3	0.2	0.7	0.2	-2.0	-2.0	0.58
MDY-E 0.1	0.1	0.9	0.9	–	–	–	–	–	–	0.74507	0.3	0.2	0.7	0.2	-2.0	-2.0	0.26

Table 5.20: Asymptotic relative efficiency with respect to the estimation of β_2 between ML Estimation for complete data and Complete Case Analysis.

5.7 Asymptotic Relative Efficiency: A Summary of Results

Estimation of β_1

Developing methods to handle missing values in the covariates one aim is to overcome the obvious inefficiency of Complete Case Analysis. The results from the comparison between ML Estimation and Complete Case Analysis in Section 5.4 demonstrate that this aim can be reached. The most impressive result about the possible gain is achieved by a comparison between ML Estimation for complete data and ML Estimation for incomplete data (Section 5.5): if the second covariate has no influence ($\beta_2 = 0$) and the covariates are uncorrelated ($\rho = 0$), than the estimation of β_1 need not to suffer from missing values in the second covariate. Correlation between the covariates or influence of the second covariate prevent this optimal result. The magnitude of the remaining gain of ML Estimation for incomplete data compared to Complete Case Analysis can differ widely, and a fair evaluation is difficult, because also the ARE between ML Estimation for complete data and Complete Case Analysis can differ widely, and a small loss here makes a large gain of ML Estimation for incomplete data compared to Complete Case Analysis impossible. It is to be emphasized that only under the MCAR assumption the global missing rate is an indicator for the loss of efficiency due to missing values and the use of Complete Case Analysis, and that it is never an indicator for the possible gain due to replacing Complete Case Analysis by ML Estimation.

PML Estimation and Filling share with ML Estimation the observation not to suffer from missing values if $\beta_2 = 0$ and $\rho = 0$. The results of the comparisons by means of asymptotic relative efficiency for other conditions are summarized in Table 5.21. PML Estimation seems to be at least nearly as efficient as ML Estimation; especially PMLY seems to be efficient for MCAR and MDX designs, and hence uniformly better than PMLX. The loss of efficiency is so small that we have not found parameter constellations, where Complete Case Analysis is better than PMLX or PMLY. Filling seems to be as efficient as ML Estimation if the MCAR assumption holds. Otherwise, with increasing variation of the missing rates, the loss can be substantially large. We found parameter constellations where the Filling method may be worse than Complete Case Analysis (Table 5.22), but independence of the covariates may prevent this.

Estimation of β_2

Units with unobservable X_2 seem to carry no information about β_2, and hence it cannot be expected that estimates of β_2 are found, which are more accurate than the Complete Case Analysis estimate. This is corroborated by our investigations, where we have always observed an ARE of 1.0 for the estimation of β_2 between ML Estimation and Complete Case Analysis. Furthermore this implies that any method worse than ML Estimation is also worse than Complete Case Analysis; i.e., PML Estimation and the Filling method are worse than Complete Case Analysis with respect to the estimation of β_2. Especially the loss of the Filling method can be substantial (see Table 5.8).

Assumption	Ordering with respect to the asymptotic relative efficiency of the estimation of β_1
MCAR	ML = PMLY = Filling $\geq$ PMLX
MCAR $\wedge\ \beta_2 = 0$	ML = PMLY = Filling = PMLX
MDX	ML = PMLY $\geq\ \dfrac{\text{Filling}}{\text{PMLX}}$
MDX $\wedge\ \beta_2 = 0$	ML = PMLY = PMLX $\geq$ Filling
MDY $\vee$ MDXY	ML $\geq\ \dfrac{\text{Filling}}{\text{PMLY}}$
$\beta_2 = 0 \wedge \rho = 0$	ML = PMLX = PMLY = Filling

Table 5.21: Comparison of ML Estimation, PML Estimation and Filling by means of asymptotic relative efficiency with respect to the estimation of β_1 under different assumptions on the missing value mechanism, the effect of the second covariate and the correlation of the covariates. "=" indicates an ARE of 1.0, "$\geq$" indicates that the second method shows a larger variance than the first. Methods with an ARE smaller or larger than 1.0 depending on the parameter constellation are arranged one above the other.

	observability rates				parameter restrictions						minimal $ARE(\beta_1)$	parameter constellations with minimal $ARE(\beta_1)$						
	q_{01}	q_{02}	q_{11}	q_{12}	p_1	p_2	ρ	γ	β_1	β_2		p_1	p_2	ρ	γ	β_1	β_2	q^A
MDX-M	0.5	0.9	0.5	0.9	–	–	–	–	–	–	0.95984	0.2	0.2	0.8	0.5	-2.0	2.0	0.58
MDX-E	0.1	0.9	0.1	0.9	–	–	–	–	–	–	0.44624	0.2	0.2	0.8	0.5	-2.0	-2.0	0.26
MDY-M	0.5	0.5	0.9	0.9	–	–	–	–	–	–	1.00747	0.3	0.2	0.7	0.2	-2.0	2.0	0.58
MDY-E	0.1	0.1	0.9	0.9	–	–	–	–	–	–	0.66422	0.3	0.2	0.7	0.2	2.0	-2.0	0.26
MDX-M	0.5	0.9	0.5	0.9	–	–	0.0	–	–	–	1.14603	0.2	0.2	0.0	0.3	-2.0	2.0	0.58
MDX-E	0.1	0.9	0.1	0.9	–	–	0.0	–	–	–	1.34747	0.2	0.2	0.0	0.4	-2.0	2.0	0.26
MDY-M	0.5	0.5	0.9	0.9	–	–	0.0	–	–	–	1.13750	0.2	0.2	0.0	0.2	-2.0	2.0	0.58
MDY-E	0.1	0.1	0.9	0.9	–	–	0.0	–	–	–	1.15510	0.4	0.2	0.0	0.2	-2.0	2.0	0.26

Table 5.22: Asymptotic relative efficiency with respect to the estimation of β_1 between Complete Case Analysis and Filling. Results of worst case analysis.

5.8 Asymptotic Bias: Comparison of Probability Imputation, Additional Category and Omission of Covariate

From our considerations in Chapter 4 we expect a serious bias for Unconditional Probability Imputation, Additional Category and Omission of Covariate if the covariates are correlated, whereas Conditional Probability Imputation should not suffer from correlation of the covariates. The second parameter highly influencing the bias is the magnitude of β_2. This is illustrated by the following result: if $\beta_2 = 0$ then all these methods yield consistent estimates of the regression parameters. For Omission of Covariate this result is obvious; for the other methods it follows from the fact that for $\beta_2 = 0$ the expectation of $\frac{\partial}{\partial\beta}\tilde{\ell}(\beta; Y, X_1, Z_2)$ coincides for all these methods.

To demonstrate that even slight correlations between the covariates can cause a substantial bias, we consider the asymptotic bias of the estimation of β_1 as a function of the correlation for all four methods (Figure 5.1). The parameter constellation is $p_1 = 0.5$, $p_2 = 0.5$, $\gamma = 0.5$, $\beta_2 = -2.0$, and $\beta_1 = 0.0$ (upper figure) or $\beta_1 = 2.0$ (lower figure), respectively. The missing value mechanism is MCAR with an observation rate of 0.7. The following observations should be noted:

- Omission of Covariate yields the largest absolute bias (for most values of ρ).
- The bias of Additional Category and Unconditional Probability Imputation nearly agrees, and for a slight correlation of $\rho = 0.3$ we observe for both methods a bias of -0.21 if $\beta_1 = 0$ and a bias of -0.38 if $\beta_1 = 2$.
- The bias of Conditional Probability Imputation is only slightly affected by the correlation and it nearly vanishes if $\beta_1 = 0$, but it may be as large as -0.13 if $\beta_1 = 2.0$.

In Figure 5.2 the same investigations are shown for parameter constellations with maximal bias of Unconditional Probability Imputation at $\rho = 0.3$ varying p_1, p_2, γ, and β_2; similar observations can be made. These figures should be convincing enough to forbid a further recommendation of Unconditional Probability Imputation, Additional Category and Omission of Covariate, if independence of the covariates cannot be assumed. Hence we restrict our further attention to Conditional Probability Imputation.

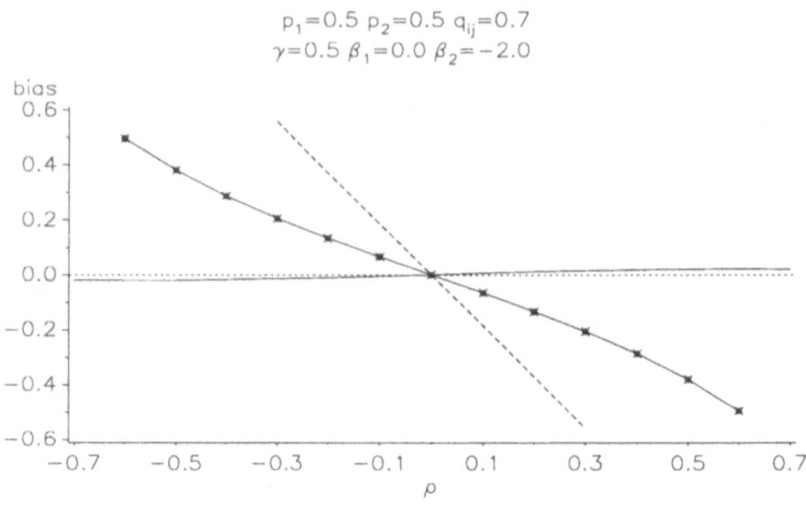

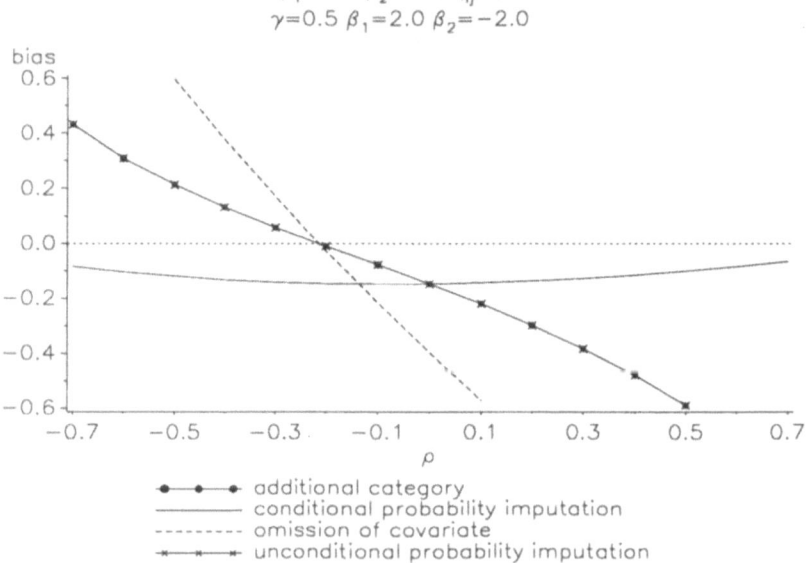

Figure 5.1: Asymptotic Bias of $\hat{\beta}_1$ for Unconditional Probability Imputation, Conditional Probability Imputation, Additional Category and Omission of Covariate

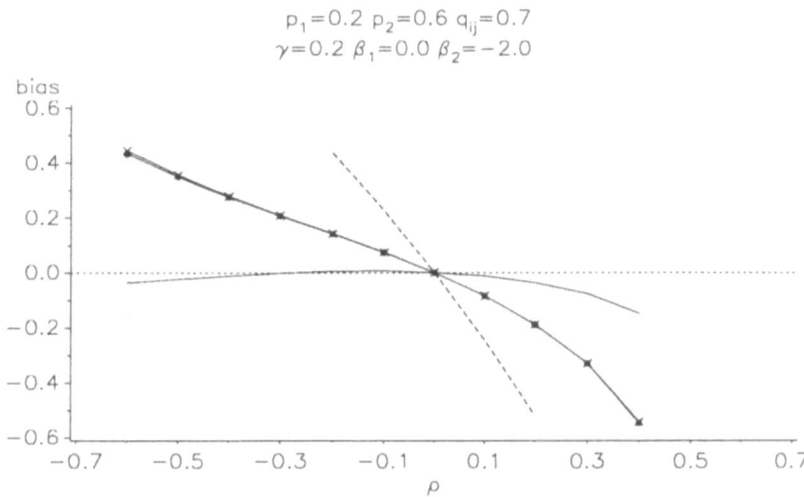

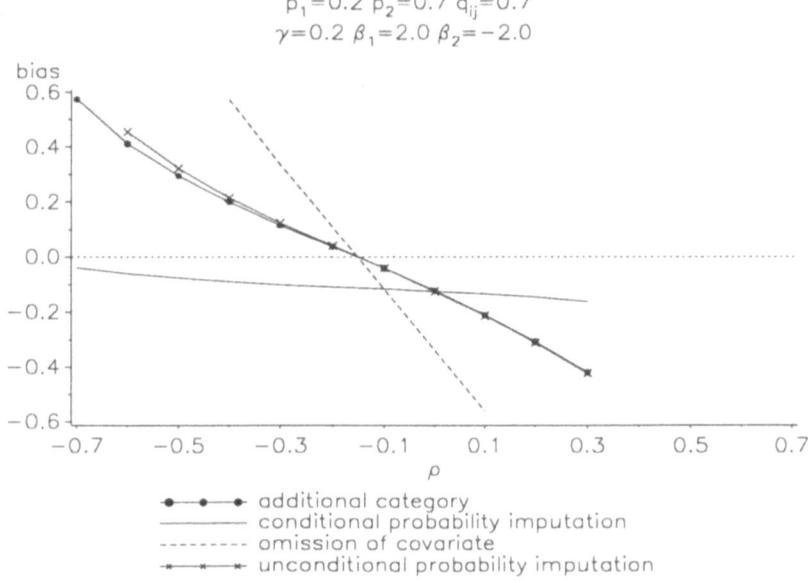

Figure 5.2: Asymptotic Bias of $\hat{\beta}_1$ for Unconditional Probability Imputation, Conditional Probability Imputation, Additional Category and Omission of Covariate

5.9 Asymptotic Bias: Evaluation of Conditional Probability Imputation

Similar to the two different estimates in the pseudo maximum likelihood approach we have also two methods of Conditional Probability Imputation, differing in the use of $\hat{\pi}$ or $\tilde{\pi}$. The choice of $\tilde{\pi}$ is necessary if we have MDY or MDXY mechanisms. Under the MDX assumption both choices are possible and result in the same asymptotic bias. Hence in this section we consider only Conditional Probability Imputation based on $\tilde{\pi}$.

In Tables 5.23 and 5.24 we show the asymptotic bias of Conditional Probability Imputation as a function of β_1 and β_2 for the six designs D1-D6. The maximal values observed may suggest to regard the bias as negligible for most constellations. The results from a worst case analysis (Tables 5.25 and 5.26) may confirm this for the moderate MCAR and MDX designs, whereas for MDY and MDXY we found parameter constellations, where Conditional Probability Imputation results in absolutely misleading estimates. Hence we have to conclude that the idea to get a close approximation to PML Estimation by Conditional Probability Imputation fails for some MDY and MDXY mechanisms. A good explanation for this failure has not yet been found; probably it is related to the observation that for these designs PML Estimation has to be regarded as a partial likelihood approach (cf. Section 4.2).

Bias is most painful if $\beta_1 = 0$, because then it may result in an erroneous postulation of an effect. In four of the six designs we have observed no asymptotic bias in the estimation of β_1 if $\beta_1 = 0$. However, the results of a worst case analysis with the restriction $\beta_1 = 0$ shows that we cannot exclude bias in general, and that this restriction also does not imply a substantial decrease of the magnitude of the worst results. The further restriction to independent covariates indicates a consistent estimation of $\beta_1 = 0$ for the MCAR and MDY designs. The key to this result is that here independence of X_1 and X_2 also implies independence of X_1 and Z_2. Then one can show that given $\beta_{1j}^0 \equiv 0$ and $\beta_{1j} \equiv 0$, the equations $E_{\beta_0} \frac{\partial}{\partial \beta_{1j}} \tilde{\ell}(\beta; Y, X_1, Z_2) = 0$ and $E_{\beta_0} \frac{\partial}{\partial \beta_0} \tilde{\ell}(\beta; Y, X_1, Z_2) = 0$ are all equivalent, i.e., there exists a solution of $E_{\beta_0} \frac{\partial}{\partial \beta} \tilde{\ell}(\beta; Y, X_1, Z_2) = 0$ with $\beta_{1j} \equiv 0$.

For biased estimates it is interesting to know whether they are always underestimating the effect of a covariate, i.e., whether they are biased to 0. However, a necessary assumption therefore is the consistency for $\beta_1 = 0$; hence a general underestimation can only occur under the MDY or MCAR assumption. The final investigation in Table 5.25 indicates that under the MDY assumption the bias can be away from zero, but the conjecture may hold under the MCAR assumption.

D1
$p_1=0.5$, $p_2=0.5$, $\rho=0.0$, $\gamma=0.5$
$q_{0j}\equiv0.7$

		β_2	
	0.0	1.0	2.0
β_1 -2.0	0.000	0.035	0.147
-1.0	0.000	0.018	0.075
0.0	0.000	0.000	0.000
1.0	0.000	-0.018	-0.075
2.0	0.000	-0.035	-0.147

D2
$p_1=0.5$, $p_2=0.5$, $\rho=0.5$, $\gamma=0.5$
$q_{0j}\equiv0.7$

			β_2		
	-2.0	-1.0	0.0	1.0	2.0
β_1 -2.0	0.119	0.027	0.000	0.026	0.101
-1.0	0.072	0.016	0.000	0.012	0.038
0.0	0.020	0.002	0.000	-0.002	-0.020
1.0	-0.038	-0.012	0.000	-0.016	-0.072
2.0	-0.101	-0.026	0.000	-0.027	-0.119

D3
$p_1=0.2$, $p_2=0.2$, $\rho=0.0$, $\gamma=0.2$
$q_{0j}\equiv0.7$

			β_2		
	-2.0	-1.0	0.0	1.0	2.0
β_1 -2.0	0.012	0.006	0.000	0.013	0.062
-1.0	0.008	0.004	0.000	0.009	0.041
0.0	0.000	0.000	0.000	0.000	0.000
1.0	-0.015	-0.006	0.000	-0.011	-0.053
2.0	-0.038	-0.014	0.000	-0.022	-0.103

D4
$p_1=0.5$, $p_2=0.5$, $\rho=0.0$, $\gamma=0.5$
$q_{i0}\equiv0.5$, $q_{i1}\equiv0.9$

		β_2	
	0.0	1.0	2.0
β_1 -2.0	0.000	0.035	0.142
-1.0	.000	0.018	0.072
0.0	0.000	0.000	0.000
1.0	0.000	-0.018	-0.072
2.0	0.000	-0.035	-0.142

D5
$p_1=0.5$, $p_2=0.5$, $\rho=0.0$, $\gamma=0.5$
$q_{0j}\equiv0.5$, $q_{1j}\equiv0.9$

		β_2	
	0.0	1.0	2.0
β_1 -2.0	0.000	0.035	0.148
-1.0	0.000	0.019	0.075
0.0	0.000	0.000	0.000
1.0	0.000	-0.019	-0.075
2.0	0.000	-0.035	-0.148

D6
$p_1=0.5$, $p_2=0.5$, $\rho=0.0$, $\gamma=0.5$
$q_{00}=0.5$, $q_{01}=0.7$, $q_{10}=0.7$, $q_{11}=0.9$

		β_2	
	0.0	1.0	2.0
β_1 -2.0	0.000	0.035	0.144
-1.0	0.000	0.018	0.072
0.0	0.000	-0.001	-0.003
1.0	0.000	-0.019	-0.077
2.0	0.000	-0.035	-0.147

Table 5.23: Asymptotic bias of $\hat{\beta}_1$ based on Conditional Probability Imputation. Note that in this table β_1 is the rowvariable and β_2 is the columnvariable.

D1

$p_1=0.5,\ p_2=0.5,\ \rho=0.0,\ \gamma=0.5$

$q_{0j}\equiv0.7$

		β_1		
		0.0	1.0	2.0
	-2.0	0.000	0.008	0.058
	-1.0	0.000	0.002	0.016
β_2	0.0	0.000	0.000	0.000
	1.0	0.000	-0.002	-0.016
	2.0	0.000	-0.008	-0.058

D2

$p_1=0.5,\ p_2=0.5,\ \rho=0.5,\ \gamma=0.5$

$q_{0j}\equiv0.7$

		β_1				
		-2.0	-1.0	0.0	1.0	2.0
	-2.0	0.047	0.016	-0.001	0.008	-0.040
	-1.0	0.006	0.002	0.000	0.001	-0.006
β_2	0.0	0.000	0.000	0.000	0.000	0.000
	1.0	-0.006	-0.001	0.000	-0.001	-0.006
	2.0	-0.040	-0.008	0.001	-0.015	-0.047

D3

$p_1=0.2,\ p_2=0.2,\ \rho=0.0,\ \gamma=0.2$

$q_{0j}\equiv0.7$

		β_1				
		-2.0	-1.0	0.0	1.0	2.0
	-2.0	0.112	0.120	0.126	0.116	0.034
	-1.0	0.010	0.011	0.012	0.011	0.039
β_2	0.0	0.000	0.000	0.000	0.000	0.000
	1.0	-0.005	-0.006	-0.006	-0.006	-0.008
	2.0	-0.034	-0.039	-0.039	-0.043	-0.061

D4

$p_1=0.5,\ p_2=0.5,\ \rho=0.0,\ \gamma=0.5$

$q_{i0}\equiv0.5,\ q_{i1}\equiv0.9$

		β_1		
		0.0	1.0	2.0
	-2.0	0.000	0.006	0.047
	-1.0	0.000	0.002	0.013
β_2	0.0	0.000	0.000	0.000
	1.0	0.000	-0.002	-0.013
	2.0	0.000	-0.006	-0.047

D5

$p_1=0.5,\ p_2=0.5,\ \rho=0.0,\ \gamma=0.5$

$q_{0j}\equiv0.5,\ q_{1j}\equiv0.9$

		β_1		
		0.0	1.0	2.0
	-2.0	-0.032	-0.008	0.049
	-1.0	-0.004	-0.001	0.007
β_2	0.0	0.000	0.000	0.000
	1.0	0.004	0.001	-0.007
	2.0	0.032	0.008	-0.049

D6

$p_1=0.5,\ p_2=0.5,\ \rho=0.0,\ \gamma=0.5$

$q_{00}=0.5,\ q_{01}=0.7,\ q_{10}=0.7,\ q_{11}=0.9$

		β_1				
		-2.0	-1.0	0.0	1.0	2.0
	-2.0	0.047	0.004	-0.007	0.014	0.058
	-1.0	0.007	0.001	-0.001	0.002	0.008
β_2	0.0	0.000	0.000	0.000	0.000	0.000
	1.0	-0.007	-0.001	0.001	-0.002	-0.008
	2.0	-0.047	-0.004	0.007	-0.014	-0.058

Table 5.24: Asymptotic bias of $\hat{\beta}_2$ based on Conditional Probability Imputation.

observability rates				parameter restrictions						maximal/ minimal $\hat{\beta}_1 - \beta_1$	parameter constellations with maximal/minimal bias						
	q_{01}	q_{02}	q_{11}	q_{12}	p_1	p_2	ρ	γ	β_1	β_2		p_1	p_2	ρ	γ	β_1	β_2	q^A
MCAR-M	0.7	0.7	0.7	0.7	–	–	–	–	–	–	0.19677	0.4	0.3	-0.5	0.8	-2.0	-2.0	0.70
											-0.19677	0.4	0.3	-0.5	0.2	2.0	-2.0	0.70
MCAR-E	0.3	0.3	0.3	0.3	–	–	–	–	–	–	0.38278	0.4	0.3	-0.5	0.8	-2.0	-2.0	0.30
											-0.38278	0.4	0.3	-0.5	0.2	2.0	-2.0	0.30
MDX-M	0.5	0.9	0.5	0.9	–	–	–	–	–	–	0.29163	0.4	0.3	-0.5	0.2	2.0	2.0	0.66
											-0.29163	0.4	0.3	-0.5	0.2	2.0	-2.0	0.66
MDX-E	0.1	0.9	0.1	0.9	–	–	–	–	–	–	0.40309	0.4	0.3	-0.5	0.8	-2.0	-2.0	0.42
											-0.40309	0.4	0.3	-0.5	0.2	2.0	2.0	0.42
MDY-M	0.5	0.5	0.9	0.9	–	–	–	–	–	–	1.64529	0.2	0.3	0.7	0.2	2.0	-2.0	0.58
											-1.64529	0.8	0.3	0.7	0.2	-2.0	-2.0	0.58
MDY-E	0.1	0.1	0.9	0.9	–	–	–	–	–	–	13.29495	0.2	0.3	0.7	0.2	0.0	-2.0	0.26
											-13.29495	0.2	0.3	0.7	0.2	0.0	-2.0	0.26
MDXY-M	0.5	0.7	0.7	0.9	–	–	–	–	–	–	0.59944	0.2	0.3	0.7	0.2	-2.0	-2.0	0.58
											-0.65914	0.8	0.3	-0.7	0.2	2.0	-2.0	0.70
MDXY-E	0.1	0.5	0.5	0.9	–	–	–	–	–	–	4.08274	0.2	0.3	0.7	0.3	2.0	-2.0	0.30
											-2.99062	0.8	0.3	-0.7	0.2	-1.0	-2.0	0.50
MCAR-M	0.7	0.7	0.7	0.7	–	–	–	–	0.0	–	0.12781	0.3	0.4	-0.5	0.8	0.0	-2.0	0.70
											-0.12781	0.3	0.4	-0.5	0.2	0.0	2.0	0.70
MCAR-E	0.3	0.3	0.3	0.3	–	–	–	–	0.0	–	0.25269	0.3	0.4	-0.5	0.8	0.0	-2.0	0.30
											-0.25269	0.3	0.4	-0.5	0.2	0.0	2.0	0.30
MDX-M	0.5	0.9	0.5	0.9	–	–	–	–	0.0	–	0.20876	0.3	0.4	-0.5	0.8	0.0	-2.0	0.62
											-0.20876	0.3	0.4	-0.5	0.2	0.0	2.0	0.62
MDX-E	0.1	0.9	0.1	0.9	–	–	–	–	0.0	–	0.30019	0.3	0.4	-0.5	0.8	0.0	-2.0	0.34
											-0.30019	0.3	0.4	-0.5	0.2	0.0	2.0	0.34
MDY-M	0.5	0.5	0.9	0.9	–	–	–	–	0.0	–	1.48693	0.2	0.3	0.7	0.2	0.0	-2.0	0.58
											-1.48693	0.8	0.3	-0.7	0.2	0.0	-2.0	0.58
MDY-E	0.1	0.1	0.9	0.9	–	–	–	–	0.0	–	13.29495	0.2	0.3	0.7	0.2	0.0	-2.0	0.26
											-13.29495	0.2	0.3	0.7	0.2	0.0	-2.0	0.26
MDXY-M	0.5	0.7	0.7	0.9	–	–	–	–	0.0	–	0.50334	0.2	0.3	0.7	0.2	0.0	-2.0	0.58
											-0.58820	0.8	0.3	-0.7	0.2	0.0	-2.0	0.70
MDXY-E	0.1	0.5	0.5	0.9	–	–	–	–	0.0	–	2.30919	0.2	0.3	0.7	0.2	0.0	-2.0	0.26
											-2.96644	0.8	0.3	-0.7	0.2	0.0	-2.0	0.50

Table 5.25: Asymptotic bias of $\hat{\beta}_1$ based on Conditional Probability Imputation. Results of worst case analysis.

observability rates				parameter restrictions						maximal/minimal $\hat{\beta}_1 - \beta_1$	parameter constellations with maximal/minimal bias						
q_{01}	q_{02}	q_{11}	q_{12}	p_1	p_2	ρ	γ	β_1	β_2		p_1	p_2	ρ	γ	β_1	β_2	q^A
MCAR-M 0.7	0.7	0.7	0.7	–	–	0.0	–	0.0	–	0.00000	all						
MCAR-E 0.3	0.3	0.3	0.3	–	–	0.0	–	0.0	–	0.00000	all						
MDX-M 0.5	0.9	0.5	0.9	–	–	0.0	–	0.0	–	0.11256	0.8	0.4	0.0	0.2	0.0	-2.0	0.82
										-0.11256	0.8	0.4	0.0	0.2	0.0	2.0	0.82
MDX-E 0.1	0.9	0.1	0.9	–	–	0.0	–	0.0	–	0.22346	0.8	0.5	0.0	0.8	0.0	-2.0	0.74
										-0.22346	0.8	0.5	0.0	0.2	0.0	-2.0	0.74
MDY-M 0.5	0.5	0.9	0.9	–	–	0.0	–	0.0	–	0.00000	all						
MDY-E 0.1	0.1	0.9	0.9	–	–	0.0	–	0.0	–	0.00000	all						
MDXY-M 0.5	0.7	0.7	0.9	–	–	0.0	–	0.0	–	0.03943	0.8	0.4	0.0	0.8	0.0	-2.0	0.82
										-0.08142	0.8	0.5	0.0	0.2	0.0	-2.0	0.72
MDXY-E 0.1	0.5	0.5	0.9	–	–	0.0	–	0.0	–	0.04967	0.8	0.3	0.0	0.8	0.0	-2.0	0.74
										-0.58116	0.2	0.2	0.0	0.2	0.0	-2.0	0.26
MCAR-M 0.7	0.7	0.7	0.7	–	–	0.0	–	≤ 0.0	–	0.14720	0.3	0.5	0.0	0.6	-2.0	-2.0	0.70
										0.00000							
MCAR-M 0.7	0.7	0.7	0.7	–	–	0.0	–	≥ 0.0	–	0.00000	many						
										-0.14720	0.3	0.5	0.0	0.4	2.0	-2.0	0.70
MCAR-E 0.3	0.3	0.3	0.3	–	–	0.0	–	≤ 0.0	–	0.30096	0.5	0.5	0.0	0.5	-2.0	-2.0	0.30
										0.00000	many						
MCAR-E 0.3	0.3	0.3	0.3	–	–	0.0	–	≥ 0.0	–	0.00000	many						
										-0.30096	0.5	0.5	0.0	0.5	2.0	-2.0	0.30
MDY-M 0.5	0.5	0.9	0.9	–	–	0.0	–	≤ 0.0	–	0.21691	0.2	0.5	0.0	0.6	-2.0	-2.0	0.74
										0.00000	many						
MDY-M 0.5	0.5	0.9	0.9	–	–	0.0	–	≥ 0.0	–	0.00000	many						
										-0.21693	0.8	0.5	0.0	0.6	2.0	-2.0	0.74
MDY-E 0.1	0.1	0.9	0.9	–	–	0.0	–	≤ 0.0	–	0.36236	0.6	0.2	0.0	0.3	-2.0	-2.0	0.34
										-0.03931	0.8	0.3	0.0	0.5	-2.0	-2.0	0.50
MDY-E 0.1	0.1	0.9	0.9	–	–	0.0	–	≥ 0.0	–	0.03931	0.2	0.3	0.0	0.5	2.0	-2.0	0.50
										-0.36236	0.4	0.2	0.0	0.3	2.0	-2.0	0.34

Table 5.25(continued): Asymptotic bias of $\hat{\beta}_1$ based on Conditional Probability Imputation. Results of worst case analysis.

observability rates				parameter restrictions						maximal/ minimal $\hat{\beta}_2 - \beta_2$	parameter constellations with maximal/minimal bias						
	q_{01}	q_{02}	q_{11}	q_{12}	p_1	p_2	ρ	γ	β_1	β_2		p_1	p_2	ρ	γ	β_1	β_2	q^A
MCAR-M	0.7	0.7	0.7	0.7	–	–	–	–	–	–	0.21060	0.4	0.3	-0.5	0.2	2.0	-2.0	0.70
											-0.21060	0.4	0.3	-0.5	0.8	-2.0	-2.0	0.70
MCAR-E	0.3	0.3	0.3	0.3	–	–	–	–	–	–	0.38798	0.4	0.3	-0.5	0.2	2.0	-2.0	0.30
											-0.38798	0.4	0.3	-0.5	0.8	-2.0	-2.0	0.30
MDX-M	0.5	0.9	0.5	0.9	–	–	–	–	–	–	0.28582	0.3	0.3	-0.4	0.8	2.0	-2.0	0.62
											-0.28582	0.3	0.3	-0.4	0.2	-2.0	2.0	0.62
MDX-E	0.1	0.9	0.1	0.9	–	–	–	–	–	–	0.32441	0.3	0.3	-0.4	0.2	1.0	-2.0	0.34
											-0.32441	0.3	0.3	-0.4	0.8	-1.0	2.0	0.34
MDY-M	0.5	0.5	0.9	0.9	–	–	–	–	–	–	4.52895	0.2	0.8	-0.6	0.2	-2.0	2.0	0.58
											-4.52895	0.2	0.2	0.6	0.2	-2.0	-2.0	0.58
MDY-E	0.1	0.1	0.9	0.9	–	–	–	–	–	–	42.82500	0.2	0.2	0.8	0.2	-2.0	2.0	0.26
											-42.82500	0.2	0.8	-0.8	0.2	-2.0	2.0	0.26
MDXY-M	0.5	0.7	0.7	0.9	–	–	–	–	–	–	1.11967	0.2	0.8	-0.5	0.2	-2.0	2.0	0.58
											-1.11967	0.2	0.2	0.5	0.2	-2.0	-2.0	0.58
MDXY-E	0.1	0.5	0.5	0.9	–	–	–	–	–	–	13.85878	0.2	0.8	-0.7	0.2	-2.0	2.0	0.26
											-13.85878	0.2	0.2	0.7	0.2	-2.0	-2.0	0.26

Table 5.26: Asymptotic bias of $\hat{\beta}_2$ based on Conditional Probability Imputation. Results of worst case analysis.

5.10 Evaluating the Underestimation of Variance of Conditional Probability Imputation

The asymptotic bias of Conditional Probability Imputation is only one problem, the other is the underestimation of variance as described in Section 4.6. By comparison with the asymptotic variance

$$I_{\beta\beta}^{ML}(\xi^0)^{-1} + I_{\beta\beta}^{ML}(\xi^0)^{-1} I_{\beta\pi}^{ML}(\xi^0) \Sigma_{\hat{\pi}^n}(\xi^0) I_{\beta\pi}^{ML}(\xi^0)' I_{\beta\beta}^{ML}(\xi^0)^{-1}$$

of the pseudo maximum likelihood estimate, we have to conclude that estimating the variance after imputation of conditional probabilities approximates only $I_{\beta\beta}^{ML}(\xi^0)^{-1}$ whereas the second term is neglected. The portion of this second term at the variance of the pseudo maximum likelihood estimate can regarded as an indicator for the magnitude of underestimation of variance after imputation of conditional probabilities.

We restrict our investigation of the magnitude of the portion of variance correction for the pseudo maximum likelihood estimate to MCAR and MDX missing value mechanisms, because we have seen in the last section that Conditional Probability Imputation cannot be recommended if an MDY or MDXY mechanism is given. In Table 5.27 the portion of variance correction with respect to the estimation of the variance of $\hat{\beta}_1$ is shown for the designs D1 to D4. The maximal value observed is 0.048.

<table>
<tr><td colspan="4" align="center">D1
$p_1=0.5$, $p_2=0.5$, $\rho=0.0$, $\gamma=0.5$
$q_{0j}\equiv0.7$</td></tr>
<tr><td></td><td colspan="3" align="center">β_1</td></tr>
<tr><td></td><td>0.0</td><td>1.0</td><td>2.0</td></tr>
<tr><td>0.0</td><td>0.000</td><td>0.000</td><td>0.000</td></tr>
<tr><td>β_2 1.0</td><td>0.007</td><td>0.007</td><td>0.005</td></tr>
<tr><td>2.0</td><td>0.023</td><td>0.020</td><td>0.015</td></tr>
</table>

<table>
<tr><td colspan="6" align="center">D2
$p_1=0.5$, $p_2=0.5$, $\rho=0.5$, $\gamma=0.5$
$q_{0j}\equiv0.7$</td></tr>
<tr><td></td><td>-2.0</td><td>-1.0</td><td>0.0</td><td>1.0</td><td>2.0</td></tr>
<tr><td></td><td colspan="5" align="center">β_1</td></tr>
<tr><td>-2.0</td><td>0.018</td><td>0.017</td><td>0.013</td><td>0.008</td><td>0.005</td></tr>
<tr><td>-1.0</td><td>0.004</td><td>0.004</td><td>0.004</td><td>0.003</td><td>0.002</td></tr>
<tr><td>β_2 0.0</td><td>0.000</td><td>0.000</td><td>0.000</td><td>0.000</td><td>0.000</td></tr>
<tr><td>1.0</td><td>0.002</td><td>0.003</td><td>0.004</td><td>0.004</td><td>0.004</td></tr>
<tr><td>2.0</td><td>0.005</td><td>0.005</td><td>0.013</td><td>0.017</td><td>0.018</td></tr>
</table>

<table>
<tr><td colspan="6" align="center">D3
$p_1=0.2$, $p_2=0.2$, $\rho=0.0$, $\gamma=0.2$
$q_{0j}=0.7$</td></tr>
<tr><td></td><td colspan="5" align="center">β_1</td></tr>
<tr><td></td><td>-2.0</td><td>-1.0</td><td>0.0</td><td>1.0</td><td>2.0</td></tr>
<tr><td>-2.0</td><td>0.001</td><td>0.003</td><td>0.005</td><td>0.007</td><td>0.010</td></tr>
<tr><td>-1.0</td><td>0.001</td><td>0.001</td><td>0.002</td><td>0.003</td><td>0.003</td></tr>
<tr><td>β_2 0.0</td><td>0.000</td><td>0.000</td><td>0.000</td><td>0.000</td><td>0.000</td></tr>
<tr><td>1.0</td><td>0.001</td><td>0.003</td><td>0.004</td><td>0.005</td><td>0.004</td></tr>
<tr><td>2.0</td><td>0.007</td><td>0.913</td><td>0.017</td><td>0.016</td><td>0.012</td></tr>
</table>

<table>
<tr><td colspan="4" align="center">D4
$p_1=0.5$, $p_2=0.5$, $\rho=0.0$, $\gamma=0.5$
$q_{i0}\equiv0.5$, $q_{i1}\equiv0.9$</td></tr>
<tr><td></td><td colspan="3" align="center">β_1</td></tr>
<tr><td></td><td>0.0</td><td>1.0</td><td>2.0</td></tr>
<tr><td>0.0</td><td>0.000</td><td>0.000</td><td>0.000</td></tr>
<tr><td>β_2 1.0</td><td>0.015</td><td>0.014</td><td>0.011</td></tr>
<tr><td>2.0</td><td>0.048</td><td>0.042</td><td>0.031</td></tr>
</table>

Table 5.27: Portion of variance correction at the variance of $\hat{\beta}_1$ of PML estimation

Results from a worst case analysis in Table 5.28 show that only for the extreme designs the portion becomes substantially large. Interestingly, the parameter constellations where the worst results occur do not show extreme values; especially they occur in the case of independence of the covariates.

With respect to the variance of $\hat{\beta}_2$ the correction does not contribute to the variance as shown in Table 5.29.

Our investigation suggests that for many constellations the underestimation of variance may be negligible. We will investigate this further in Section 6.3.

observability rates				parameter restrictions						maximal portion of correction	parameter constellations with maximal correction						
q_{01}	q_{02}	q_{11}	q_{12}	p_1	p_2	ρ	γ	β_1	β_2		p_1	p_2	ρ	γ	β_1	β_2	q^A
MCAR-M	0.7	0.7	0.7	0.7	–	–	–	–	–	–	0.02255	–	0.5	0.0	0.5	0.0	-2.0	0.70
MCAR-E	0.3	0.3	0.3	0.3	–	–	–	–	–	–	0.24387	–	0.5	0.0	0.5	0.0	-2.0	0.30
MDX-M	0.5	0.9	0.5	0.9	–	–	–	–	–	–	0.07141	0.8	0.5	0.0	0.5	0.0	-2.0	0.82
MDX-E	0.1	0.9	0.1	0.9	–	–	–	–	–	–	0.58269	0.8	0.5	0.0	0.5	0.0	-2.0	0.74

Table 5.28: Portion of variance correction at the variance of $\hat{\beta}_1$ of PML estimation

observability rates				parameter restrictions						maximal portion of correction	parameter constellations with maximal correction						
q_{01}	q_{02}	q_{11}	q_{12}	p_1	p_2	ρ	γ	β_1	β_2		p_1	p_2	ρ	γ	β_1	β_2	q^A
MCAR-M	0.7	0.7	0.7	0.7	–	–	–	–	–	–	0.00000	all						
MCAR-E	0.3	0.3	0.3	0.3	–	–	–	–	–	–	0.00000	all						
MDX-M	0.5	0.9	0.5	0.9	–	–	–	–	–	–	0.00000	all						
MDX-E	0.1	0.9	0.1	0.9	–	–	–	–	–	–	0.00000	all						

Table 5.29: Portion of variance correction at the variance of $\hat{\beta}_2$ of PML estimation

5.11 The Importance of the Variance Correction for the Filling Method

In Section 4.3 we have shown that the variance estimate of the Filling method can be regarded as a correction of the naive variance estimate from the filled table. It may raise the question whether this correction is negligible. Asymptotically, the ratio between the uncorrected and corrected variance is equal to the ARE between ML Estimation for complete data and Filling. Hence from our considerations in Section 5.7 we know with respect to the estimation of β_1 that this ratio is equal to 1.0 if $\beta_2 = 0.0$ and $\rho = 0.0$. Otherwise the ratio must be smaller than the ARE between ML Estimation for complete data and ML Estimation for incomplete data, because the Filling method is less efficient than the latter. Hence from this comparison (Section 5.5) we already know that the variance correction can be substantial. The values in Table 5.30 corroborate this.

With respect to the estimation of β_2 we can conclude with the help of similar arguments that the ratio between corrected and uncorrected variance is equal to the observation rate in MCAR designs. Hence with increasing missing rate the correction becomes more and more substantial.

D1 $p_1{=}0.5$, $p_2{=}0.5$, $\rho{=}0.0$, $\gamma{=}0.5$ $q_{0j}{\equiv}0.7$				
		β_1		
		0.0	1.0	2.0
	0.0	1.000	1.000	1.000
β_2	1.0	0.975	0.971	0.961
	2.0	0.916	0.906	0.883

D2 $p_1{=}0.5$, $p_2{=}0.5$, $\rho{=}0.5$, $\gamma{=}0.5$ $q_{0j}{\equiv}0.7$						
				β_1		
		-2.0	-1.0	0.0	1.0	2.0
	-2.0	0.931	0.901	0.861	0.821	0.791
	-1.0	0.946	0.920	0.891	0.864	0.841
β_2	0.0	0.903	0.903	0.903	0.903	0.903
	1.0	0.841	0.864	0.891	0.920	0.946
	2.0	0.791	0.821	0.861	0.901	0.931

D3 $p_1{=}0.2$, $p_2{=}0.2$, $\rho{=}0.0$, $\gamma{=}0.2$ $q_{0j}{\equiv}0.7$						
				β_1		
		-2.0	-1.0	0.0	1.0	2.0
	-2.0	0.996	0.991	0.983	0.973	0.959
	-1.0	0.998	0.996	0.993	0.989	0.983
β_2	0.0	1.000	1.000	1.000	1.000	1.000
	1.0	0.994	0.989	0.986	0.982	0.975
	2.0	0.966	0.950	0.940	0.931	0.916

D4 $p_1{=}0.5$, $p_2{=}0.5$, $\rho{=}0.0$, $\gamma{=}0.5$ $q_{i0}{\equiv}0.5$, $q_{i1}{\equiv}0.9$				
			β_1	
		0.0	1.0	2.0
	0.0	1.000	1.000	1.000
β_2	1.0	0.968	0.963	0.950
	2.0	0.894	0.882	0.854

D5 $p_1{=}0.5$, $p_2{=}0.5$, $\rho{=}0.0$, $\gamma{=}0.5$ $q_{0j}{\equiv}0.5$, $q_{1j}{\equiv}0.9$				
			β_1	
		0.0	1.0	2.0
	0.0	1.000	1.000	1.000
β_2	1.0	0.968	0.963	0.950
	2.0	0.894	0.882	0.854

D6 $p_1{=}0.5$, $p_2{=}0.5$, $\rho{=}0.0$, $\gamma{=}0.5$ $q_{00}{=}0.5$, $q_{01}{=}0.7$, $q_{10}{=}0.7$, $q_{11}{=}0.9$						
				β_1		
		-2.0	-1.0	0.0	1.0	2.0
	0.0	1.000	1.000	1.000	1.000	1.000
β_2	1.0	0.951	0.964	0.971	0.969	0.960
	2.0	0.855	0.887	0.905	0.901	0.882

Table 5.30: Asymptotic ratio between uncorrected and corrected variance estimates for the variance of $\hat{\beta}_1$ of the Filling method

6. Quantitative Comparisons: Results of Finite Sample Size Simulation Studies

The investigations of the last chapter were based on asymptotic arguments. It remains to show that the results of the comparisons are transferable to the finite sample size. Moreover, the properties of the methods themselves have been examined so far only asymptotically, and the estimation of variance is also based on asymptotic results.

In the first section of this chapter we investigate properties of the consistent estimation methods (ML Estimation, PML Estimation and Filling) for the finite sample size. The aim is to demonstrate that these methods work well with respect to unbiasedness and validity of confidence intervals. As we have to expect small deviations of the bias from 0 and of the coverage probability of the confidence intervals from their nominal level, we include Complete Case Analysis in our examination, so that we can regard the deviations as acceptable, if they are not larger than those of Complete Case Analysis.

The comparison of the power to detect an effect $\beta_1 \neq 0$ with these methods is the topic of the second section. Here the major aim is to establish the gain in power in comparison with Complete Case Analysis.

The third section considers the finite properties of Conditional Probability Imputation. Here our interests concern the consequences of asymptotic bias and underestimation of the asymptotic variance for the finite sample size situation.

All examinations for finite sample sizes are based on simulation studies. We restrict our investigation to the case of two dichotomous covariates and we use the same parametrization as in the last chapter. We will also refer to some of the special parameter constellations D1-D6 used there. For each parameter constellation considered we create 2500 data sets of size n, and apply the methods to them, i.e. results for different methods but the same parameter constellation are based on an identical sequence of data sets. For the investigations of an estimate $\hat{\beta}_i$ the following statistics were computed and appear in the representations of the results:

bias: The average difference between the estimates and the true parameter.

cvg: The relative frequency to find the true parameter within the 95% confidence interval. This is an approximation to the true coverage probability of the confidence interval. The limits of the confidence interval are computed as $\hat{\beta}_i \pm 1.96 \widehat{Var}(\hat{\beta}_i)$ and the variance is estimated as described for each method in Chapter 4.

pow: The relative frequency to find 0 outside of the 95% confidence interval for β_1. This is an approximation to the power of the associated test to reject the null hypothesis $\beta_1 = 0$.

It is well known that ML estimates for the parameters of a logistic regression model need not to exist, if in some of the strata defined by the combination of the categories of the covariates the outcome variable shows no variation. Hence we cannot exclude that for some of our data sets our estimation procedure fails. This may have also other reasons, e.g. in the PML Estimation procedure the computation of the estimates of the nuisance parameters can result in a division by 0. We try to choose the sample size n always so large that the number of failures of the estimation procedure is less than 25 (i.e., 1% of all data sets); exceptions are indicated in the tables. The reported relative frequencies are always based on the total number of data sets with success of the estimation procedure.

The choice of 2500 repetitions in the simulation study implies that the standard error of the estimated coverage probability of the 95% confidence interval is less than 0.005 and that the standard error of the estimated power is less than 0.01.

For the computation of the estimates we always used the scoring variant of the Newton-Raphson method. No EM algorithm was used. The initial value for the regression parameters is 0.0. For the computation of the ML estimates the initial value of $\pi_{k|j}$ is $\frac{1}{K}$. Convergence was assumed, if the maximal absolute difference between two consecutive parameter values was less than 10^{-8}. The maximal number of iterations was 25.

6.1 Finite Behavior of ML Estimation, PML Estimation, Filling and Complete Case Analysis

We start our investigation for the parameter constellation of the design D1. In Table 6.1 estimates of the bias of $\hat{\beta}_1$ and the coverage probability of the 95% confidence interval for β_1 are shown for the following five methods: ML Estimation, the two variants of PML Estimation, Filling and Complete Case Analysis. The results for the first four methods are very similar; differences only concern the third decimal digit. Contrary, the bias of Complete Case Analysis is often distinctly larger. Although the coverage probabilities are only estimated, we observe very few values less than 0.95, so that we can conclude that the confidence intervals are slightly conservative.

The investigation of the parameter constellations D2 and D3 in Tables 6.2 and 6.3 allow similar observations; only for the design D2 with correlated covariates we cannot regard the confidence intervals as conservative.

The fourth investigation is based on the parameter constellation of the design D6 (Table 6.4. As we have here an MDXY missing value mechanism, the variant PMLX of PML Estimation is not applicable, and the estimates of Complete Case Analysis are asymptotically biased. We can observe this bias also in the finite sample size situation; the bias of the other methods is distinctly smaller. The results for ML Estimation, PML Estimation and Filling are again very similar, but Filling shows an increased bias for some constellation.

One may argue that the finite behavior of the methods may break down for parameter constellations with extreme differences in the missing rates. Hence we investigate at least one such constellation; we chose an extreme MDY mechanism with missing rates of 0.1 and 0.9, and the other parameters are chosen such that they cover a constellation with minimal asymptotic relative efficiency with respect to the estimation of β_1 between ML Estimation and Filling (cf. Table 5.7). We have to choose a sample size of $n = 600$ in order get enough executable data sets for our study. Again the violations are of similar magnitude for all methods, but note that the bias of Filling exceeds for some constellations the bias of Complete Case Analysis.

$p_1 = 0.5, p_2 = 0.5, \rho = 0.0, \gamma = 0.5, q_{ij} \equiv 0.7, n = 150$											
		ML		PMLX		PMLY		Filling		CC	
β_1	β_2	bias	cvg	bias	cvg	bias	cvg	bias	cvg	bias	cvg
-2.0	-2.0	-0.098	0.968	-0.092	0.968	-0.098	0.968	-0.098	0.968	-0.121	0.968
-2.0	-1.0	-0.068	0.951	-0.066	0.951	-0.067	0.951	-0.068	0.952	-0.095	0.954
-2.0	0.0	-0.060	0.947	-0.060	0.947	-0.060	0.947	-0.061	0.946	-0.083	0.950
-2.0	1.0	-0.073	0.954	-0.071	0.953	-0.073	0.955	-0.074	0.955	-0.094	0.946
-2.0	2.0	-0.106	0.971	-0.100	0.968	-0.105	0.971	-0.106	0.971	-0.122	0.964
-1.0	-2.0	-0.043	0.960	-0.040	0.962	-0.043	0.960	-0.042	0.960	-0.056	0.956
-1.0	-1.0	-0.031	0.954	-0.030	0.954	-0.031	0.954	-0.031	0.953	-0.044	0.945
-1.0	0.0	-0.030	0.956	-0.030	0.956	-0.030	0.956	-0.030	0.956	-0.042	0.954
-1.0	1.0	-0.036	0.956	-0.035	0.955	-0.036	0.956	-0.037	0.955	-0.049	0.955
-1.0	2.0	-0.055	0.954	-0.052	0.954	-0.055	0.954	-0.055	0.955	-0.068	0.953
0.0	-2.0	0.002	0.957	0.002	0.957	0.002	0.957	0.002	0.956	0.001	0.954
0.0	-1.0	-0.003	0.951	-0.003	0.951	-0.003	0.950	-0.003	0.950	-0.007	0.954
0.0	0.0	-0.007	0.950	-0.007	0.950	-0.007	0.950	-0.007	0.949	-0.014	0.950
0.0	1.0	-0.011	0.958	-0.010	0.958	-0.011	0.958	-0.011	0.958	-0.019	0.956
0.0	2.0	-0.016	0.960	-0.015	0.961	-0.016	0.961	-0.016	0.962	-0.024	0.956
1.0	-2.0	0.046	0.957	0.044	0.957	0.046	0.957	0.047	0.956	0.052	0.956
1.0	-1.0	0.027	0.952	0.026	0.952	0.027	0.952	0.027	0.953	0.030	0.956
1.0	0.0	0.017	0.955	0.017	0.955	0.017	0.955	0.017	0.955	0.016	0.948
1.0	1.0	0.014	0.954	0.014	0.954	0.014	0.953	0.014	0.952	0.011	0.957
1.0	2.0	0.023	0.956	0.021	0.956	0.023	0.956	0.023	0.956	0.017	0.958
2.0	-2.0	0.085	0.964	0.080	0.964	0.085	0.964	0.086	0.964	0.093	0.964
2.0	-1.0	0.067	0.958	0.066	0.958	0.067	0.959	0.068	0.959	0.077	0.959
2.0	0.0	0.051	0.952	0.051	0.952	0.051	0.952	0.051	0.952	0.059	0.954
2.0	1.0	0.053	0.958	0.052	0.958	0.053	0.958	0.054	0.957	0.055	0.963
2.0	2.0	0.073	0.959	0.069	0.958	0.073	0.959	0.074	0.958	0.072	0.963

Table 6.1: Comparison of Maximum Likelihood Estimation, Pseudo Maximum Likelihood Estimation, Filling and Complete Case Analysis: Bias and Coverage Probability of the Estimation of β_1. Results of a Monte Carlo Study.

$p_1 = 0.5, p_2 = 0.5, \rho = 0.5, \gamma = 0.5, q_{ij} \equiv 0.7, n = 225$											
		ML		PMLX		PMLY		Filling		CC	
β_1	β_2	bias	cvg	bias	cvg	bias	cvg	bias	cvg	bias	cvg
-2.0	-2.0	-0.035	0.948	-0.034	0.948	-0.035	0.948	-0.035	0.948	-0.056	0.951
-2.0	-1.0	-0.036	0.949	-0.036	0.950	-0.035	0.948	-0.036	0.949	-0.054	0.955
-2.0	0.0	-0.056	0.957	-0.055	0.954	-0.056	0.957	-0.056	0.957	-0.072	0.953
-2.0	1.0	-0.076	0.962	-0.074	0.960	-0.076	0.962	-0.077	0.961	-0.086	0.961
-2.0	2.0	-0.101	0.965	-0.096	0.964	-0.101	0.965	-0.101	0.964	-0.107	0.969
-1.0	-2.0	0.000	0.951	-0.001	0.952	0.000	0.952	0.000	0.952	-0.014	0.960
-1.0	-1.0	-0.014	0.947	-0.015	0.948	-0.014	0.947	-0.013	0.948	-0.026	0.956
-1.0	0.0	-0.023	0.954	-0.023	0.953	-0.023	0.954	-0.023	0.953	-0.032	0.952
-1.0	1.0	-0.045	0.950	-0.043	0.950	-0.045	0.950	-0.046	0.951	-0.051	0.956
-1.0	2.0	-0.070	0.962	-0.065	0.958	-0.070	0.962	-0.070	0.962	-0.072	0.960
0.0	-2.0	0.024	0.950	0.021	0.952	0.024	0.951	0.025	0.950	0.013	0.956
0.0	-1.0	0.011	0.953	0.009	0.954	0.011	0.952	0.011	0.953	0.005	0.957
0.0	0.0	-0.003	0.948	-0.003	0.948	-0.003	0.949	-0.003	0.948	-0.007	0.952
0.0	1.0	-0.016	0.952	-0.014	0.952	-0.016	0.952	-0.016	0.952	-0.019	0.954
0.0	2.0	-0.036	0.960	-0.033	0.960	-0.036	0.961	-0.036	0.960	-0.035	0.955
1.0	-2.0	0.063	0.964	0.059	0.966	0.063	0.964	0.064	0.965	0.057	0.962
1.0	-1.0	0.034	0.952	0.032	0.954	0.034	0.953	0.035	0.952	0.031	0.956
1.0	0.0	0.020	0.956	0.020	0.956	0.020	0.956	0.020	0.956	0.018	0.956
1.0	1.0	0.008	0.953	0.010	0.953	0.008	0.953	0.008	0.954	0.009	0.952
1.0	2.0	0.003	0.959	0.005	0.959	0.003	0.959	0.003	0.958	0.009	0.954
2.0	-2.0	0.097	0.970	0.093	0.971	0.097	0.970	0.099	0.970	0.094	0.972
2.0	-1.0	0.072	0.964	0.069	0.964	0.072	0.964	0.073	0.964	0.070	0.956
2.0	0.0	0.045	0.956	0.045	0.955	0.046	0.956	0.046	0.956	0.050	0.950
2.0	1.0	0.038	0.950	0.040	0.950	0.038	0.950	0.039	0.950	0.049	0.947
2.0	2.0	0.035	0.957	0.035	0.957	0.035	0.956	0.036	0.957	0.049	0.949

Table 6.2: Comparison of Maximum Likelihood Estimation, Pseudo Maximum Likelihood Estimation, Filling and Complete Case Analysis: Bias and Coverage Probability of the Estimation of β_1. Results of a Monte Carlo Study.

$p_1 = 0.2, p_2 = 0.2, \rho = 0.0, \gamma = 0.2, q_{ij} \equiv 0.7, n = 400$											
		ML		PMLX		PMLY		Filling		CC	
β_1	β_2	bias	cvg	bias	cvg	bias	cvg	bias	cvg	bias	cvg
-2.0	-2.0	*-0.077*	*0.963*	*-0.106*	*0.964*	*-0.056*	*0.962*	*-0.056*	*0.962*	*-0.045*	*0.965*
-2.0	-1.0	*-0.068*	*0.963*	*-0.095*	*0.964*	*-0.041*	*0.962*	*-0.041*	*0.962*	*-0.027*	*0.962*
-2.0	0.0	*-0.091*	*0.968*	*-0.110*	*0.969*	*-0.055*	*0.966*	*-0.055*	*0.966*	*-0.038*	*0.968*
-2.0	1.0	*-0.098*	*0.966*	*-0.108*	*0.967*	*-0.055*	*0.964*	*-0.056*	*0.964*	*-0.042*	*0.965*
-2.0	2.0	*-0.125*	*0.960*	*-0.126*	*0.960*	*-0.083*	*0.958*	*-0.084*	*0.958*	*-0.084*	*0.959*
-1.0	-2.0	*-0.066*	*0.956*	*-0.068*	*0.955*	*-0.064*	*0.957*	*-0.064*	*0.957*	*-0.085*	*0.965*
-1.0	-1.0	-0.066	0.955	-0.068	0.955	-0.066	0.955	-0.066	0.956	-0.095	0.966
-1.0	0.0	-0.071	0.958	-0.074	0.958	-0.070	0.958	-0.070	0.958	-0.093	0.967
-1.0	1.0	-0.082	0.954	-0.082	0.955	-0.076	0.957	-0.077	0.957	-0.102	0.962
-1.0	2.0	-0.071	0.958	-0.070	0.959	-0.070	0.960	-0.070	0.960	-0.091	0.959
0.0	-2.0	*-0.024*	*0.954*	*-0.024*	*0.954*	*-0.024*	*0.955*	*-0.024*	*0.955*	*-0.033*	*0.956*
0.0	-1.0	-0.020	0.952	-0.020	0.952	-0.020	0.952	-0.020	0.952	-0.029	0.958
0.0	0.0	-0.026	0.954	-0.026	0.954	-0.026	0.954	-0.026	0.954	-0.035	0.960
0.0	1.0	-0.025	0.958	-0.025	0.958	-0.025	0.958	-0.025	0.959	-0.031	0.953
0.0	2.0	-0.029	0.952	-0.028	0.953	-0.029	0.952	-0.029	0.952	-0.037	0.957
1.0	-2.0	*0.001*	*0.959*	*0.000*	*0.959*	*0.001*	*0.959*	*0.001*	*0.959*	*0.000*	*0.953*
1.0	-1.0	0.003	0.957	0.002	0.957	0.003	0.957	0.003	0.956	0.001	0.950
1.0	0.0	0.004	0.950	0.004	0.950	0.004	0.950	0.004	0.950	0.003	0.953
1.0	1.0	0.003	0.956	0.003	0.955	0.003	0.957	0.003	0.957	0.000	0.952
1.0	2.0	0.003	0.954	0.003	0.954	0.003	0.954	0.003	0.954	0.003	0.950
2.0	-2.0	*0.017*	*0.949*	*0.016*	*0.947*	*0.017*	*0.949*	*0.017*	*0.948*	*0.022*	*0.952*
2.0	-1.0	0.022	0.950	0.022	0.951	0.022	0.950	0.022	0.950	0.027	0.951
2.0	0.0	0.021	0.954	0.021	0.954	0.021	0.954	0.021	0.954	0.025	0.952
2.0	1.0	0.022	0.950	0.022	0.949	0.022	0.950	0.022	0.950	0.026	0.956
2.0	2.0	0.023	0.945	0.021	0.946	0.023	0.945	0.023	0.946	0.026	0.947

Table 6.3: Comparison of Maximum Likelihood Estimation, Pseudo Maximum Likelihood Estimation, Filling and Complete Case Analysis: Bias and Coverage Probability of the Estimation of β_1. Results of a Monte Carlo Study. Numbers in italic indicate results with more than 25 non-executable data sets within the 2500 Monte Carlo repetitions.

| $p_1 = 0.5$, $p_2 = 0.5$, $\rho = 0.0$, $\gamma = 0.5$, $q_{01} = 0.5$, $q_{02} = 0.7$, $q_{11} = 0.7$, $q_{12} = 0.9$, $n = 150$ | | | | | | | | |
| | | ML | | PMLY | | Filling | | CC | |
β_1	β_2	bias	cvg	bias	cvg	bias	cvg	bias	cvg
-2.0	-2.0	-0.105	0.965	-0.104	0.964	-0.113	0.970	-0.211	0.953
-2.0	-1.0	-0.081	0.960	-0.081	0.961	-0.084	0.962	-0.189	0.955
-2.0	0.0	-0.071	0.950	-0.072	0.950	-0.076	0.950	-0.180	0.942
-2.0	1.0	-0.082	0.960	-0.083	0.959	-0.087	0.960	-0.180	0.954
-2.0	2.0	-0.108	0.957	-0.108	0.957	-0.119	0.964	-0.198	0.962
-1.0	-2.0	-0.057	0.960	-0.057	0.959	-0.059	0.965	-0.152	0.956
-1.0	-1.0	-0.045	0.952	-0.044	0.953	-0.046	0.953	-0.141	0.942
-1.0	0.0	-0.040	0.952	-0.040	0.952	-0.042	0.951	-0.132	0.944
-1.0	1.0	-0.050	0.960	-0.050	0.960	-0.054	0.961	-0.139	0.953
-1.0	2.0	-0.060	0.964	-0.060	0.964	-0.066	0.964	-0.147	0.955
0.0	-2.0	-0.017	0.953	-0.017	0.953	-0.018	0.953	-0.097	0.948
0.0	-1.0	-0.018	0.956	-0.018	0.955	-0.018	0.956	-0.099	0.947
0.0	0.0	-0.022	0.956	-0.022	0.956	-0.023	0.956	-0.105	0.948
0.0	1.0	-0.024	0.956	-0.025	0.956	-0.026	0.955	-0.105	0.952
0.0	2.0	-0.022	0.960	-0.022	0.960	-0.026	0.960	-0.100	0.944
1.0	-2.0	0.024	0.961	0.025	0.962	0.025	0.963	-0.047	0.954
1.0	-1.0	0.008	0.958	0.009	0.958	0.009	0.958	-0.066	0.950
1.0	0.0	0.004	0.957	0.004	0.957	0.004	0.956	-0.074	0.952
1.0	1.0	0.010	0.958	0.010	0.958	0.009	0.958	-0.065	0.949
1.0	2.0	0.020	0.963	0.019	0.963	0.018	0.963	-0.055	0.953
2.0	-2.0	0.070	0.964	0.070	0.965	0.072	0.964	0.003	0.953
2.0	-1.0	0.040	0.959	0.040	0.958	0.040	0.958	-0.030	0.948
2.0	0.0	0.038	0.958	0.038	0.957	0.038	0.957	-0.031	0.946
2.0	1.0	0.051	0.958	0.050	0.958	0.050	0.958	-0.018	0.952
2.0	2.0	0.069	0.965	0.068	0.966	0.068	0.964	-0.003	0.960

Table 6.4: Comparison of Maximum Likelihood Estimation, Pseudo Maximum Likelihood Estimation, Filling and Complete Case Analysis: Bias and Coverage Probability of the Estimation of β_1. Results of a Monte Carlo Study.

$p_1 = 0.4,\ p_2 = 0.3,\ \rho = 0.6,\ \gamma = 0.5,\ q_{i1} \equiv 0.1,\ q_{i2} \equiv 0.9,\ n = 600$									
		ML		PMLY		Filling		CC	
β_1	β_2	bias	cvg	bias	cvg	bias	cvg	bias	cvg
-2.0	-2.0	-0.034	0.960	-0.035	0.962	-0.038	0.963	-0.045	0.955
-2.0	-1.0	-0.041	0.960	-0.051	0.962	-0.072	0.968	-0.055	0.958
-2.0	0.0	-0.040	0.961	-0.063	0.965	-0.127	0.974	-0.051	0.963
-2.0	1.0	-0.051	0.955	-0.067	0.958	-0.179	0.962	-0.057	0.956
-2.0	2.0	-0.078	0.969	-0.090	0.967	-0.259	0.959	-0.077	0.968
-1.0	-2.0	0.013	0.959	0.019	0.961	0.024	0.962	0.007	0.953
-1.0	-1.0	0.011	0.959	0.010	0.964	0.011	0.968	0.003	0.958
-1.0	0.0	-0.011	0.961	-0.017	0.967	-0.035	0.974	-0.017	0.957
-1.0	1.0	-0.020	0.956	-0.028	0.951	-0.077	0.965	-0.016	0.951
-1.0	2.0	-0.042	0.953	-0.049	0.949	-0.133	0.960	-0.042	0.958
0.0	-2.0	0.051	0.957	0.056	0.958	0.075	0.959	0.045	0.967
0.0	-1.0	0.034	0.951	0.038	0.954	0.056	0.958	0.039	0.953
0.0	0.0	0.011	0.948	0.013	0.952	0.016	0.957	0.009	0.951
0.0	1.0	0.001	0.951	-0.004	0.952	-0.021	0.958	0.012	0.953
0.0	2.0	-0.012	0.956	-0.019	0.955	-0.061	0.967	0.007	0.954
1.0	-2.0	0.092	0.958	*0.094*	*0.955*	0.145	0.956	0.098	0.961
1.0	-1.0	0.059	0.963	0.066	0.961	0.104	0.962	0.068	0.960
1.0	0.0	0.020	0.950	0.027	0.955	0.050	0.966	0.028	0.960
1.0	1.0	0.013	0.951	0.015	0.952	0.024	0.957	0.036	0.957
1.0	2.0	0.004	0.949	-0.001	0.948	-0.016	0.952	0.033	0.947
2.0	-2.0	*0.097*	*0.962*	*0.095*	*0.963*	*0.176*	*0.962*	*0.100*	*0.976*
2.0	-1.0	0.086	0.956	*0.091*	*0.955*	0.154	0.953	0.106	0.972
2.0	0.0	0.059	0.960	0.065	0.966	0.108	0.969	0.082	0.959
2.0	1.0	0.024	0.958	0.028	0.955	0.055	0.963	0.069	0.946
2.0	2.0	0.027	0.951	0.028	0.955	0.043	0.958	0.061	0.949

Table 6.5: Comparison of Maximum Likelihood Estimation, Pseudo Maximum Likelihood Estimation, Filling and Complete Case Analysis: Bias and Coverage Probability of the Estimation of β_1. Results of a Monte Carlo Study. Numbers in italic indicate results with more than 25 non-executable data sets within the 2500 Monte Carlo repetitions.

6.2 Power Comparisons

We start our power comparisons with the three designs D1, D2 and D3. (Table 6.6 - 6.8). We consider the power to detect the alternative $\beta_1 = 1$ or $\beta_1 = -1$ varying β_2. The differences between the power of ML Estimation, PML Estimation and Filling are only marginal, but the gain compared to Complete Case Analysis is distinct. The gain is larger for D1 and D3 compared to D2, which coincides with the asymptotic considerations of the last chapter (cf. Table 5.11).

The possible loss of PML Estimation and Filling in comparison with ML Estimation is demonstrated in Table 6.9. The parameter constellation coincides with the last one of the last section, i.e., the ARE between ML Estimation and Filling is small. The results for the finite sample size show that the power of both PMLY and Filling is smaller than the power of ML Estimation, and the loss is more distinct for Filling than for PMLY. But the power of all methods is distinctly larger than the power of Complete Case Analysis.

\multicolumn{7}{c}{$p_1 = 0.5,\ p_2 = 0.5,\ \rho = 0.0,\ \gamma = 0.5,\ q_{ij} \equiv 0.7,\ n = 150$}						
		ML	PMLX	PMLY	Filling	CC
β_1	β_2	pow	pow	pow	pow	pow
-1.0	-2.0	0.721	0.718	0.721	0.722	0.607
-1.0	-1.0	0.823	0.822	0.823	0.823	0.693
-1.0	0.0	0.855	0.855	0.854	0.854	0.718
-1.0	1.0	0.815	0.815	0.815	0.815	0.693
-1.0	2.0	0.707	0.705	0.708	0.709	0.612
1.0	-2.0	0.725	0.725	0.725	0.726	0.612
1.0	-1.0	0.816	0.816	0.816	0.816	0.682
1.0	0.0	0.838	0.838	0.838	0.838	0.698
1.0	1.0	0.804	0.805	0.804	0.803	0.671
1.0	2.0	0.715	0.716	0.712	0.713	0.574

Table 6.6: Comparison of Maximum Likelihood Estimation, Pseudo Maximum Likelihood Estimation, Filling and Complete Case Analysis: Power in detecting $\beta_1 \neq 0$ with a test based on the 95% confidence interval. Results of a Monte Carlo Study.

$p_1 = 0.5$, $p_2 = 0.5$, $\rho = 0.5$, $\gamma = 0.5$, $q_{ij} \equiv 0.7$, $n = 225$						
		ML	PMLX	PMLY	Filling	CC
β_1	β_2	pow	pow	pow	pow	pow
-1.0	-2.0	0.768	0.772	0.768	0.770	0.692
-1.0	-1.0	0.850	0.851	0.849	0.850	0.751
-1.0	0.0	0.856	0.856	0.856	0.857	0.763
-1.0	1.0	0.823	0.824	0.824	0.823	0.736
-1.0	2.0	0.716	0.714	0.716	0.716	0.622
1.0	-2.0	0.714	0.710	0.713	0.716	0.627
1.0	-1.0	0.817	0.815	0.816	0.818	0.710
1.0	0.0	0.860	0.860	0.860	0.858	0.756
1.0	1.0	0.842	0.842	0.842	0.842	0.736
1.0	2.0	0.772	0.770	0.770	0.771	0.670

Table 6.7: Comparison of Maximum Likelihood Estimation, Pseudo Maximum Likelihood Estimation, Filling and Complete Case Analysis: Power in detecting $\beta_1 \neq 0$ with a test based on the 95% confidence interval. Results of a Monte Carlo Study.

$p_1 = 0.2$, $p_2 = 0.2$, $\rho = 0.0$, $\gamma = 0.2$, $q_{ij} \equiv 0.7$, $n = 400$						
		ML	PMLX	PMLY	Filling	CC
β_1	β_2	pow	pow	pow	pow	pow
-1.0	-2.0	0.764	0.766	0.764	0.762	0.578
-1.0	-1.0	0.773	0.772	0.772	0.772	0.582
-1.0	0.0	0.775	0.776	0.774	0.774	0.589
-1.0	1.0	0.763	0.763	0.763	0.765	0.590
-1.0	2.0	0.703	0.702	0.703	0.703	0.570
1.0	-2.0	0.913	0.914	0.913	0.912	0.798
1.0	-1.0	0.922	0.922	0.922	0.922	0.811
1.0	0.0	0.930	0.930	0.930	0.930	0.826
1.0	1.0	0.913	0.912	0.912	0.912	0.803
1.0	2.0	0.856	0.856	0.856	0.855	0.753

Table 6.8: Comparison of Maximum Likelihood Estimation, Pseudo Maximum Likelihood Estimation, Filling and Complete Case Analysis: Power in detecting $\beta_1 \neq 0$ with a test based on the 95% confidence interval. Results of a Monte Carlo Study.

$p_1 = 0.4, p_2 = 0.3, \rho = 0.6, \gamma = 0.3, n = 600$					
$q_{i1} \equiv 0.1, q_{i2} \equiv 0.9$					
		ML	PMLY	Filling	CC
β_1	β_2	pow	pow	pow	pow
-1.0	-2.0	0.758	0.724	0.714	0.563
-1.0	-1.0	0.809	0.786	0.780	0.590
-1.0	0.0	0.845	0.831	0.835	0.617
-1.0	1.0	0.815	0.790	0.763	0.574
-1.0	2.0	0.747	0.722	0.523	0.532
1.0	-2.0	0.760	*0.706*	0.643	0.519
1.0	-1.0	0.845	0.825	0.804	0.576
1.0	0.0	0.882	0.860	0.862	0.589
1.0	1.0	0.898	0.869	0.849	0.615
1.0	2.0	0.869	0.827	0.746	0.598

Table 6.9: Comparison of Maximum Likelihood Estimation, Pseudo Maximum Likelihood Estimation, Filling and Complete Case Analysis: Power in detecting $\beta_1 \neq 0$ with a test based on the 95% confidence interval. Results of a Monte Carlo Study.

6.3 Evaluation of Conditional Probability Imputation

Our considerations in Section 5.10 about the underestimation of the asymptotic variance using Conditional Probability Imputation suggest that this effect is maximal in the case of uncorrelated covariates and a balanced distribution of X_2. In Table 6.10 we consider for such a situation the bias and coverage probability with respect to the estimation of β_1. We consider three MCAR designs with varying missing rates and two MDX designs. Let us first look at the results if $\beta_1 = 0$. As shown in Section 5.9 the asymptotic bias vanishes under the MCAR assumption. Indeed, the finite bias is negligible for all designs. However, if β_2 is large and the observation rates are small, then the coverage probabilities of the confidence intervals are distinctly smaller than 0.95. This effect is only due to underestimation of variance. Contrary, if $\beta_1 \neq 0$ coverage probabilities are too small even for large observation rates, but this is always accompanied by a distinct bias.

Our second investigation aims at the consequence of asymptotic bias, which is most harmful if $\beta_1 = 0$. In Table 6.11 we consider the parameter constellation with maximal asymptotic bias in the estimation of β_1 given $\beta_1 = 0$ (cf. Table 5.25). Indeed, we observe also for the finite sample size a distinct biased estimation of β_1 if β_2 is large, and the bias increases with increasing missing rate. However, with one exception this bias does not result in a violation of the coverage probability of the 95% confidence interval; probably biased estimates are accompanied with an overestimation of the variance. So it remains unclear whether the bias of Conditional Probability Imputation may really result in the erroneous establishing of an effect.

$p_1 = 0.5, p_2 = 0.5, \rho = 0.0, \gamma = 0.5, n = 150$											
		$q_{ij} \equiv 0.7$		$q_{ij} \equiv 0.5$		$q_{ij} \equiv 0.3$		$q_{i1} \equiv 0.5$ $q_{i2} \equiv 0.9$		$q_{i1} \equiv 0.1$ $q_{i2} \equiv 0.9$	
β_1	β_2	bias	cvg	bias	cvg	bias	cvg	bias	cvg	bias	cvg
-2.0	-2.0	0.084	0.939	0.211	0.889	0.264	0.843	0.073	0.942	0.176	0.843
-2.0	-1.0	-0.020	0.942	0.042	0.944	0.032	0.948	-0.028	0.957	0.028	0.931
-2.0	0.0	-0.051	0.946	-0.012	0.956	-0.050	0.960	-0.062	0.950	-0.036	0.952
-2.0	1.0	-0.017	0.950	0.043	0.948	0.024	0.946	-0.035	0.953	0.014	0.932
-2.0	2.0	0.088	0.940	0.208	0.893	0.248	0.851	0.060	0.944	0.150	0.835
-1.0	-2.0	0.047	0.949	0.125	0.925	0.143	0.884	0.037	0.948	0.106	0.857
-1.0	-1.0	-0.007	0.951	0.041	0.947	0.024	0.943	-0.017	0.954	0.020	0.926
-1.0	0.0	-0.026	0.956	0.008	0.955	-0.021	0.950	-0.036	0.953	-0.009	0.953
-1.0	1.0	-0.009	0.954	0.042	0.949	0.019	0.936	-0.025	0.953	0.011	0.925
-1.0	2.0	0.043	0.945	0.125	0.914	0.128	0.891	0.018	0.940	0.085	0.848
0.0	-2.0	0.003	0.949	0.032	0.935	0.016	0.909	-0.013	0.953	0.013	0.854
0.0	-1.0	-0.002	0.949	0.030	0.952	0.011	0.940	-0.015	0.951	0.010	0.930
0.0	0.0	-0.007	0.950	0.033	0.957	0.007	0.948	-0.022	0.953	0.004	0.952
0.0	1.0	-0.009	0.956	0.030	0.944	0.006	0.938	-0.026	0.954	0.001	0.917
0.0	2.0	-0.011	0.952	0.031	0.938	-0.000	0.911	-0.031	0.944	-0.003	0.852
1.0	-2.0	-0.043	0.946	-0.060	0.927	-0.109	0.887	-0.058	0.946	-0.076	0.850
1.0	-1.0	0.003	0.951	0.024	0.943	-0.004	0.941	-0.013	0.950	-0.008	0.933
1.0	0.0	0.014	0.955	0.053	0.945	0.034	0.952	0.001	0.956	0.015	0.954
1.0	1.0	-0.009	0.949	0.023	0.942	-0.015	0.939	-0.021	0.954	-0.015	0.924
1.0	2.0	-0.063	0.937	-0.063	0.926	-0.128	0.895	-0.072	0.939	-0.092	0.846
2.0	-2.0	-0.092	0.936	-0.147	0.910	-0.228	0.852	-0.098	0.930	-0.154	0.834
2.0	-1.0	0.018	0.955	0.032	0.943	-0.009	0.941	-0.001	0.952	-0.017	0.932
2.0	0.0	0.043	0.949	0.085	0.949	0.059	0.949	0.030	0.957	0.035	0.950
2.0	1.0	0.004	0.952	0.028	0.953	-0.020	0.934	-0.004	0.952	-0.024	0.927
2.0	2.0	-0.106	0.926	-0.152	0.914	-0.251	0.852	-0.113	0.930	-0.168	0.830

Table 6.10: Evaluation of Conditional Probability Imputation: Bias and Coverage Probability of the Estimation of β_1. Results of a Monte Carlo Study.

$p_1 = 0.3,\ p_2 = 0.4,\ \rho = -0.5,\ \gamma = 0.8,\ n = 200$									
		$q_{ij} \equiv 0.7$		$q_{ij} \equiv 0.5$		$q_{ij} \equiv 0.3$		$q_{i1} \equiv 0.5$ $q_{i2} \equiv 0.9$		$q_{i1} \equiv 0.1$ $q_{i2} \equiv 0.9$	
β_1	β_2	bias	cvg	bias	cvg	bias	cvg	bias	cvg	bias	cvg
0.0	-2.0	0.156	0.969	0.279	0.962	0.270	0.951	0.235	0.960	0.293	0.921
0.0	-1.0	0.042	0.961	0.075	0.961	0.068	0.955	0.063	0.960	0.079	0.950
0.0	0.0	0.016	0.958	0.026	0.962	0.014	0.958	0.017	0.958	0.039	0.960
0.0	1.0	0.026	0.958	0.048	0.958	0.047	0.960	0.041	0.956	0.122	0.961
0.0	2.0	0.053	0.951	0.094	0.955	0.112	0.956	0.094	0.952	0.263	0.965

Table 6.11: Evaluation of Conditional Probability Imputation: Bias and Coverage Probability of the Estimation of β_1. Results of a Monte Carlo Study.

7. Examples

So far our investigations have pointed out a lot of strengths and weaknesses of the considered methods. We want to illustrate some of these features by comparing the results of different methods applied to the same data set. We start with some artificially generated data sets, where we know the missing value mechanism, and then we present an example with a real data set. For all examples we consider the following ten different methods described in Chapter 4:

- Maximum Likelihood Estimation (ML)
- Pseudo Maximum Likelihood Estimation with

    - estimation of π by $\hat{\pi}^n$ (PMLX)
    - estimation of π by $\tilde{\pi}^n$ (PMLY)

- the Filling method
- Complete Case Analysis (CC)
- Additional Category (AC)
- Conditional Probability Imputation with

    - estimation of π by $\hat{\pi}^n$ (CPI)
    - estimation of π by $\tilde{\pi}^n$ (CPIY)

- Unconditional Probability Imputation (UPI)
- Omission of Covariate (OC)

7.1 Illustrating Artificial Examples

Our examples are based on an artificial data set (Table 7.1) used by Breslow & Day (1980, p. 102) to demonstrate the effect of confounding. The distributions of both covariates are balanced; the empirical correlation is 0.4. ML estimates for the regression parameters based on the complete data yields $\hat{\beta}_{12} = 2.20$ and $\hat{\beta}_{22} = -1.02$. We now generate from the complete data new data sets with missing values in X_2 according to a pregiven missing value mechanism.

	$X_1 = 1$		$X_1 = 2$	
	$X_2 = 1$	$X_2 = 2$	$X_2 = 1$	$X_2 = 2$
$Y = 0$	90	50	10	50
$Y = 1$	50	10	50	90

Table 7.1: Artificial data set

We start with an MCAR mechanism with an observation probability of 0.7. The created data set, estimates of the regression parameters, and estimates of their standard deviations resulting from the application of the ten different methods are shown in Table 7.2. The last row includes the complete data estimates for the purpose of comparison. ML Estimation, both variants of PML Estimation and Filling give identical results, and the estimates of the regression parameters coincide with the estimates from the complete data. Complete Case Analysis yields the same estimates for the regression parameters, but the estimate for β_{12} shows a larger standard deviation than the other methods according to the inefficiency of Complete Case Analysis. Due to the correlation of the covariates the bias of Additional Category and Unconditional Probability Imputation is much larger than the bias of Conditional Probability Imputation, and the bias of Omission of Covariate is the largest. The bias is always accompanied with an underestimation of variance, which is especially distinct for Additional Category and Unconditional Probability Imputation, where the estimated standard deviations of $\hat{\beta}_{12}$ are smaller than the corresponding estimates in the complete data case.

	$X_1 = 1$				$X_1 = 2$			
	$Z_2 = 1$	$Z_2 = 2$	$Z_2 =?$	observation rate	$Z_2 = 1$	$Z_2 = 2$	$Z_2 =?$	observation rate
$Y = 0$	63	35	42	0.7	7	35	28	0.7
$Y = 1$	35	7	28	0.7	35	63	42	0.7

	$\hat{\beta}_{12}$	$\widehat{\text{sdv}}(\hat{\beta}_{12})$	$\hat{\beta}_{22}$	$\widehat{\text{sdv}}(\hat{\beta}_{22})$
ML	2.20	0.296	-1.02	0.328
PMLX	2.20	0.296	-1.02	0.328
PMLY	2.20	0.296	-1.02	0.328
Filling	2.20	0.296	-1.02	0.328
CC	2.20	0.328	-1.02	0.328
AC	2.00	0.251	-0.91	0.297
CPI	2.16	0.280	-1.01	0.324
CPIY	2.16	0.280	-1.01	0.324
UPI	2.00	0.251	-0.91	0.297
OC	1.70	0.218	–	–
complete data	2.20	0.275	-1.02	0.275

Table 7.2: Artificial data set generated from the complete data set of Table 7.1 according to an MCAR missing value mechanism with observation probability $q = 0.7$ and results from the application of ten different methods.

In the second example we consider an MCAR mechanism with an observation probability of $q = 0.3$ (Table 7.3). The observations are similar, but all differences are more distinct. Note that the estimated standard deviations of Additional Category and Unconditional Probability Imputation now suggest a more precise estimation of $\hat{\beta}_{12}$ than in the first example, although the missing rate is now much larger. The estimated standard deviations of Conditional Probability Imputation seem now to be substantially too small, which agrees with our considerations in Section 6.3.

	$X_1 = 1$				$X_1 = 2$			
	$Z_2 = 1$	$Z_2 = 2$	$Z_2 =?$	observation rate	$Z_2 = 1$	$Z_2 = 2$	$Z_2 =?$	observation rate
$Y = 0$	27	15	98	0.3	3	15	42	0.3
$Y = 1$	15	3	42	0.3	15	27	98	0.3

	$\hat{\beta}_{12}$	$\widehat{sdv}(\hat{\beta}_{12})$	$\hat{\beta}_{22}$	$\widehat{sdv}(\hat{\beta}_{22})$
ML	2.20	0.375	-1.02	0.502
PMLX	2.20	0.375	-1.02	0.502
PMLY	2.20	0.375	-1.02	0.502
Filling	2.20	0.375	-1.02	0.502
CC	2.20	0.502	-1.02	0.502
AC	1.81	0.230	-0.91	0.413
CPI	2.13	0.311	-1.01	0.487
CPIY	2.13	0.311	-1.01	0.487
UPI	1.81	0.230	-0.91	0.413
OC	1.70	0.218	–	–
complete data	2.20	0.275	-1.02	0.275

Table 7.3: Artificial data set generated from the complete data set of Table 7.1 according to an MCAR missing value mechanism with observation probability $q = 0.3$ and results from the application of ten different methods.

In the third example (Table 7.4) we generate the missing values according to an MDXY missing value mechanism with observation rates $q_{01} = 0.5$, $q_{02} = 0.7$, $q_{11} = 0.7$, and $q_{12} = 0.9$, i.e., it coincides with the moderate MDXY missing value mechanism considered in the last two chapters. Now we can observe a slight difference between the two variants of PML Estimation, because the estimation of π in the PMLX variant is inappropriate. Filling, ML Estimation and PMLY agree. Complete Case Analysis shows a biased estimate $\hat{\beta}_{12}$, which is due to the variation of the missing rates (cf. Section 4.4). The bias of Additional Category is for both regression parameters now larger than the bias of Unconditional Probability Imputation. Again the bias is accompanied with small standard deviations compared to the complete data estimates. Similar to the variants of PML Estimation, we observe also different results for the two variants of Conditional Probability Imputation.

	$X_1 = 1$				$X_1 = 2$			
	$Z_2 = 1$	$Z_2 = 2$	$Z_2 =?$	observation rate	$Z_2 = 1$	$Z_2 = 2$	$Z_2 =?$	observation rate
$Y = 0$	45	25	70	0.5	7	35	18	0.7
$Y = 1$	35	7	18	0.7	45	81	14	0.9

	$\hat{\beta}_{12}$	$\widehat{sdv}(\hat{\beta}_{12})$	$\hat{\beta}_{22}$	$\widehat{sdv}(\hat{\beta}_{22})$
ML	2.20	0.296	-1.02	0.331
PMLX	2.19	0.296	-1.01	0.328
PMLY	2.20	0.296	-1.02	0.331
Filling	2.20	0.296	-1.02	0.332
CC	2.11	0.332	-1.02	0.331
AC	1.77	0.257	-0.83	0.296
CPI	2.16	0.280	-0.99	0.324
CPIY	2.16	0.280	-1.01	0.324
UPI	2.01	0.251	-0.96	0.298
OC	1.70	0.218	–	–
complete data	2.20	0.275	-1.02	0.275

Table 7.4: Artificial data set generated from the complete data set of Table 7.1 according to an MDXY missing value mechanism with observation probabilities $q_{01} = 0.5$, $q_{02} = 0.7$, $q_{11} = 0.7$, and $q_{12} = 0.9$, and results from the application of ten different methods.

In the fourth example (Table 7.5) we consider an MDXY missing value mechanisms with more extreme variation between the observation rates, which coincides with the extreme MDXY missing value mechanisms considered in the last two chapters. The observations are similar to those of the preceding example, but the differences are more distinct. Additional category and Complete Case Analysis yield a larger bias then Omission of Covariate. Also the slightly smaller efficiency of Filling compared to ML Estimation is now visible in increased standard deviations for both parameters, and similar for PML Estimation of β_{22}.

	$X_1 = 1$				$X_1 = 2$			
	$Z_2 = 1$	$Z_2 = 2$	$Z_2 =?$	observation rate	$Z_2 = 1$	$Z_2 = 2$	$Z_2 =?$	observation rate
$Y = 0$	9	5	126	0.1	5	25	30	0.5
$Y = 1$	25	5	30	0.5	45	81	14	0.9

	$\hat{\beta}_{12}$	$\widehat{sdv}(\hat{\beta}_{12})$	$\hat{\beta}_{22}$	$\widehat{sdv}(\hat{\beta}_{22})$
ML	2.20	0.326	-1.02	0.428
PMLX	2.13	0.318	-0.84	0.377
PMLY	2.20	0.326	-1.02	0.435
Filling	2.20	0.329	-1.02	0.454
CC	1.18	0.452	-1.02	0.428
AC	0.88	0.289	-0.89	0.387
CPI	2.08	0.293	-0.80	0.371
CPIY	2.14	0.289	-1.01	0.381
UPI	1.94	0.240	-1.18	0.349
OC	1.70	0.218	–	–
complete data	2.20	0.275	-1.02	0.275

Table 7.5: Artificial data set generated from the complete data set of Table 7.1 according to an MDXY missing value mechanism with observation probabilities $q_{01} = 0.1$, $q_{02} = 0.5$, $q_{11} = 0.5$, and $q_{12} = 0.9$, and results from the application of ten different methods.

7.2 An Example with a Real Data Set

In this chapter we consider an example with data from a case-control study. The example arises in the "International Radiation Study on Cervical Cancer Patients", a study which investigates the relation between radiation and breast cancer risk in patients treated for cancer of the cervix (Boice et al. 1989). Estrogen replacement therapy is regarded as a potential confounder, but this variable is only known for about half of the subjects. Due to the high missing rate an examination was not presented in the original paper, first considerations are given by Blettner(1987) in her Ph.D. thesis. As shown in Table 7.6, the missing rates vary for cases and controls and, additionally, depend on the exposure to radiation.

	$Y = 0$ (controls)		$Y = 1$ (cases)	
	$X_1 = 1$ (unexposed)	$X_1 = 2$ (exposed)	$X_1 = 1$ (unexposed)	$X_1 = 2$ (exposed)
$Z_2 = 1$ (without estrogen therapy)	32	502	21	264
$Z_2 = 2$ (with estrogen therapy)	22	150	17	104
$Z_2 = ?$ (estrogen therapy unknown)	65	788	28	404
missing rate	54.6%	54.7%	42.4%	52.3%

Table 7.6: Data of the example from the "International Radiation Study on Cervical Cancer Patients"

In the following we consider the estimation of the effect of the exposure as well as of the confounder. The results of the ten methods are listed in Table 7.7, including confidence intervals. If we assume that the MAR assumption is valid, we have to regard the ML estimate as the best estimate and can compare the others estimates with it. PMLY gives the same result as ML, and also PMLX, although the missing rates suggest that we have an MDXY mechanisms

	$\hat{\beta}_{12}$	$\widehat{sdv}(\hat{\beta}_{12})$	CI	$\hat{\beta}_{22}$	$\widehat{sdv}(\hat{\beta}_{22})$	CI
ML	0.012	0.162	$-0.306 - 0.330$	0.264	0.140	$-0.011 - 0.539$
PMLX	0.012	0.162	$-0.306 - 0.331$	0.264	0.142	$-0.013 - 0.541$
PMLY	0.012	0.162	$-0.306 - 0.330$	0.264	0.140	$-0.011 - 0.539$
Filling	0.013	0.162	$-0.306 - 0.331$	0.265	0.141	$-0.010 - 0.541$
CC	-0.175	0.223	$-0.612 - 0.263$	0.263	0.140	$-0.011 - 0.539$
AC	-0.005	0.161	$-0.320 - 0.310$	0.275	0.140	$0.002 - 0.550$
CPI	0.013	0.162	$-0.304 - 0.331$	0.269	0.141	$-0.008 - 0.546$
CPIY	0.013	0.162	$-0.304 - 0.331$	0.269	0.141	$-0.008 - 0.546$
UPI	-0.009	0.161	$-0.324 - 0.305$	0.280	0.141	$0.004 - 0.556$
OC	-0.034	0.160	$-0.347 - 0.279$	–	–	–

Table 7.7: Application of ten methods to the data set of Table 7.6. Estimates of regression coefficients, estimates of standard deviation, and 95% confidence intervals.

here, but the violation of the MDX assumption is not large enough to show an effect. The result of Filling is also similar to ML; the deviation from MCAR is not large enough to decrease the accuracy of the estimate distinctly. Estimation of β_{12} by Complete Case Analysis results here in a distinct deviation from the ML estimate. This can be explained by the variation of the missing rates. The estimate of β_{12} by Conditional Probability Imputation coincides with the ML estimate, whereas the estimate of β_{22} shows a small deviation. The deviations of Unconditional Probability Imputation and Additional Category are larger, which can be explained by the correlation between exposure and confounder. The deviation of Omission of Covariate is still larger, agreeing with our results in Section 5.8. The estimates of the variance are all very similar with exception of the Complete Case Analysis.

However, the MAR assumption is questionable in this example. This will be further discussed in the next chapter.

8. Sensitivity Analysis

ML Estimation, PML Estimation and Filling are all based on the MAR assumption. In many applications this assumption is highly questionable. In general we have no chance to check the validity of the MAR assumption based on the observed contingency table: missing values in X_2 cause $2 \times J$ new cells in our contingency table, but the MAR assumption introduces already $2 \times J$ new parameters $(q_{ij})_{i=0,1;j=1,...,J}$, hence additional parameters are not identifiable [8†].

However, if we specify a non-MAR missing value mechanism with $2 \times J$ unknown parameters, it may remain possible to estimate the regression parameters of interest. Such a missing value mechanism may for example represent the assumption that subjects with $X_2 = 2$ refuse to answer twice as often as subjects with $X_2 = 1$. If we compute estimates of β under several assumptions of plausible non-MAR missing value mechanisms and if we get similar results, then we can conclude that the estimates are not sensitive against violations of the MAR assumption; if the results highly differ, we have to conclude that the missing values prevent an reasonable assessment of the effect of the covariates.

Parametrizations for non-MAR Mechanisms

If we want to estimate under a non-MAR mechanism, it is not necessary to specify the observation probabilities $(q_{ijk})_{i=0,1;j=1,...,J;k=1,...,K}$ completely. We are allowed to use up to $2 \times J$ free parameters similar as under the MAR assumption. The first parametrization considered is a multiplicative decomposition of the missingness probabilities, i.e.,

$$1 - q_{ijk} := c_{ij}c_{ijk} \quad \text{with } c_{ij1} = 1 \tag{8.1}$$

such that $c_{ijk} = \frac{1-q_{ijk}}{1-q_{ij1}}$ is the relative risk of the occurrence of a missing value for subjects with $X_2 = k$ compared to subjects with $X_2 = 1$. Now we can specify a class of non-MAR missing value mechanisms by the values $(c_{ijk})_{i=0,1;j=1,...,J;k=2,...,K}$, whereas the parameters $(c_{ij})_{i=0,1;j=1,...,J}$ are free parameters.

An alternative parametrization is based on a multiplicative decomposition of the missingness odds, i.e.,

$$\frac{1 - q_{ijk}}{q_{ijk}} = \gamma_{ij}\gamma_{ijk} \quad \text{with } \gamma_{ij1} = 1 \tag{8.2}$$

such that γ_{ijk} is the missingness odds ratio for subjects with $X_2 = k$ compared to subjects with $X_2 = 1$. $(\gamma_{ij})_{i=0,1;j=1,...,J}$ are again free parameters.

In the following we consider for both parametrizations ML Estimation, PML Estimation and the Filling method, respectively.

Maximum Likelihood Estimation

For the first parametrization, the likelihood can be maximized independently for $(c_{ij})_{i=0,1;j=1,...,J}$ and (β, π). The contribution of a single unit with $Y = y$, $X_1 = j$ and

---

[8†] Exactly, this argument is only valid, if we want to fit a saturated model to the contingency table of the complete data case. A logistic regression model with no interaction between the covariates leaves at least one degree of freedom, hence a class of non-MAR mechanism with an appropriate parametrization may be identifiable. This point is not further discussed in this book.

$Z_2 = k$ to the remaining part of the loglikelihood is

$$\ell^{ML}(\beta, \pi; y, j, k) = \begin{cases} \log[\mu_{jk}(\beta)^y(1 - \mu_{jk}(\beta))^{1-y}] + \log \pi_{k|j} & \text{if } k \neq ? \\ \log[\sum_{k=1}^{K} c_{yjk}\mu_{jk}(\beta)^y(1 - \mu_{jk}(\beta))^{1-y}\pi_{k|j}] & \text{if } k = ? \end{cases}.$$

Traditional theory yields consistency and asymptotic normality, and estimates of the variance of the regression parameter estimates can be based on the inverse of the information matrix. The EM algorithm can be used to compute the estimates of the regression parameters; compared to estimation under the MAR assumption (Section 4.1) we have only to change the meaning and computation of $r_{k|ij}(\beta, \pi)$, which is now

$$r_{k|ij}(\beta, \pi) := P_{\beta,\pi}(X_2 = k | Y = i, X_1 = j, O_2 = 0)$$

$$= \frac{c_{ijk}\pi_{k|j}\mu_{jk}(\beta)^i(1 - \mu_{jk}(\beta))^{1-i}}{\sum_{k'=1}^{K} c_{ijk'}\pi_{k'|j}\mu_{jk'}(\beta)^i(1 - \mu_{jk'}(\beta))^{1-i}}.$$

For the second parametrization a joint maximization over $((\gamma_{ij})_{i=0,1;j=1,...,J}, \beta, \pi)$ of the loglikelihood is necessary. The contribution of a single unit with $Y = y$, $X_1 = j$ and $Z_2 = k$ to the loglikelihood is

$$\ell^{ML}((\gamma_{ij})_{i=0,1;j=1,...,J}, \beta, \pi; y, j, k)$$

$$= \begin{cases} \log \frac{1}{1+\gamma_{ij}\gamma_{ijk}} + \log[\mu_{jk}(\beta)^y(1 - \mu_{jk}(\beta))^{1-y}] + \log \pi_{k|j} & \text{if } k \neq ? \\ \log[\sum_{k=1}^{K} \frac{\gamma_{ij}\gamma_{ijk}}{1+\gamma_{ij}\gamma_{ijk}}\mu_{jk}(\beta)^y(1 - \mu_{jk}(\beta))^{1-y}\pi_{k|j}] & \text{if } k = ? \end{cases}.$$

The same theoretical results as above can be applied. In the EM algorithm we now have to use the formula

$$r_{k|ij}(\beta, \pi, (\gamma_{ij})_{i=0,1;j=1,...,J}) = \frac{\frac{\gamma_{ij}\gamma_{ijk}}{1+\gamma_{ij}\gamma_{ijk}}\pi_{k|j}\mu_{jk}(\beta)^i(1 - \mu_{jk}(\beta))^{1-i}}{\sum_{k'=1}^{K} \frac{\gamma_{ij}\gamma_{ijk'}}{1+\gamma_{ij}\gamma_{ijk'}}\pi_{k'|j}\mu_{jk'}(\beta)^i(1 - \mu_{jk'}(\beta))^{1-i}}.$$

Additionally we need to compute in each step new values γ_{ij}^{t+1}. A single γ_{ij}^{t+1} results from maximizing

$$\sum_{k=1}^{K} n_{ijk} \log \frac{1}{1 + \gamma_{ij}\gamma_{ijk}} + n_{ij?}r_{k|ij}(\beta^t, \pi^t, (\gamma_{ij}^t)_{i=0,1;j=1,...,J}) \log \frac{\gamma_{ij}\gamma_{ijk}}{1 + \gamma_{ij}\gamma_{ijk}}$$

over γ_{ij}. The solution of this maximization task requires an iterative procedure.

Pseudo Maximum Likelihood Estimation

Here this approach is not very interesting, because we cannot estimate π from the distribution of the covariates alone. A possible solution results from the use of the filled table described in the next subsection to achieve an estimate for π.

Filling

Here it is the task to find a simple formula to construct a table $(\hat{n}_{ijk}^*)_{i=0,1;j=1,...,J;k=1,...,K}$ such that the relative cell frequencies are consistent estimates for the true cell probabilities $(p_{ijk}^0)_{i=0,1;j=1,...,J;k=1,...,K}$. In general we can achieve such a table by dividing n_{ijk} by q_{ijk}. Replacing q_{ijk} according to the chosen parametrization, it remains to find simple estimates for the unknown parameters $(c_{ij})_{i=0,1;j=1,...,J}$ or $(\gamma_{ij})_{i=0,1;j=1,...,J}$, respectively. These can be achieved by requiring $\hat{n}_{ij.}^* = n_{ij.}$, which leads to

$$\hat{c}_{ij} := \frac{n_{ijk}/c_{ijk}}{n_{ij.}} \quad \text{and} \quad \hat{\gamma}_{ij} := \frac{n_{ij?}}{\sum_{k=1}^{K}\gamma_{ijk}n_{ijk}}$$

such that the entries of the reconstructed table are

$$\hat{n}_{ijk}^* := n_{ij.}\frac{n_{ijk}/c_{ijk}}{\sum_{k'=1}^{K}n_{ijk'}/c_{ijk'}}$$

and

$$\hat{n}_{ijk}^* := n_{ijk} + n_{ij?}\frac{n_{ijk}\gamma_{ijk}}{\sum_{k'=1}^{K}n_{ijk'}\gamma_{ijk'}} \quad 9\dagger) \ .$$

For the second parametrization the technique can be regarded as distributing the units with a missing value to the cells of completely observed units. Analyzing the new tables with logistic regression gives consistent estimates of the regression parameters. Similar as under the MAR assumption the asymptotic variance of the regression parameter estimates can be achieved. For the second parametrization explicit formulas are given in Appendix B.4.

The Choice of Parametrization

So far we have considered two possible ways to specify a non-MAR mechanism. Considering ML estimation specification by missingness relative risks has the clear advantage that no additional parameters have to be estimated. Contrary, specification by missingness odds ratios results in a natural generalization of the Filling method. However, we should ask which type of specification is more appropriate from the statistical point of view. If all missing rates are small the difference between relative risks and odds ratios is small. However, if the missing rates are highly varying in dependence of Y and X_1 relative risks are no good idea to represent a common change of missing rates. You have to take into account that there may be subgroups with a vary low missing rate, say 0.1, and simultaneously other subgroups with a high missing rate, say 0.6.

Example of a Sensitivity Analysis

In the example from the case-control study considered in the last chapter the MAR assumption is highly questionable. It is probable that an estrogen replacement therapy when given is better documented than when it is not given. A sensitivity analysis can examine, whether such a violation has a high impact on the resulting estimates. In the following we use the parametrization (8.2).

$9\dagger$) The resulting relative cell frequencies are also ML estimates for the cell probabilities under a multinomial model.

γ_2	β_{12}	CI	β_{22}	CI
0.2	0.0042	-0.312 – 0.320	0.296	0.034 – 0.558
0.3	0.0068	-0.310 – 0.323	0.291	0.026 – 0.557
0.4	0.0087	-0.308 – 0.326	0.287	0.018 – 0.556
0.5	0.0101	-0.307 – 0.328	0.282	0.012 – 0.554
0.6	0.0111	-0.307 – 0.329	0.279	0.006 – 0.552
0.7	0.0118	-0.306 – 0.330	0.275	0.001 – 0.550
0.8	0.0123	-0.306 – 0.331	0.272	-0.003 – 0.547
0.9	0.0125	-0.306 – 0.331	0.269	-0.007 – 0.544
1.0	0.0126	-0.306 – 0.331	0.265	-0.010 – 0.541
1.2	0.0123	-0.307 – 0.331	0.259	-0.016 – 0.535
1.4	0.0118	-0.307 – 0.331	0.254	-0.021 – 0.528
1.6	0.0109	-0.308 – 0.330	0.248	-0.025 – 0.521
1.8	0.0100	-0.309 – 0.329	0.243	-0.029 – 0.515
2.0	0.0089	-0.310 – 0.328	0.240	-0.033 – 0.508
2.5	0.0061	-0.313 – 0.325	0.226	-0.040 – 0.493
3.0	0.0033	-0.315 – 0.322	0.216	-0.049 – 0.478
4.0	-0.0016	-0.319 – 0.316	0.198	-0.056 – 0.451
5.0	-0.0057	-0.323 – 0.311	0.183	-0.063 – 0.429

Table 8.1: Sensitivity analysis under the assumption of a constant missingness odds ratio for cases/controls and exposed/unexposed subjects. Estimates of regression coefficients and 95% confidence intervals based on the Filling method.

In a first step we assume that the missingness odds ratio does not vary between cases and controls and between exposed and unexposed subjects, i.e. $\gamma_{ij2} \equiv: \gamma_2$, where γ_2 is the missingness odds ratio of subjects with estrogen replacement therapy compared to subjects without. This does not imply that we have the same missing rates for cases and controls as well as for exposed and unexposed subjects, this type of variation continues to be modeled by the free parameters $(\gamma_{ij})_{i=0,1;j=1,...,J}$.

In Table 8.1 we examine the variation of the estimated regression coefficients and their confidence intervals dependent on γ_2. The variation of β_{12} seems to be negligible, especially for $\gamma_2 \leq 1$, which corresponds to the probable situation of better documentation for a given therapy than for a non-given. The variation of β_{22} is much higher, and for small values of γ_2 the effect becomes significant at the 5%-level.

One may conjecture that an estimated effect of nearly 0.0 is never sensitive against violations of the MAR assumption. This is not true in general, as demonstrated in Table 8.2, where we assume differences of the missingness odds ratio between cases and controls, exposed and unexposed, and both, respectively. However, it is rather unlikely that these estimates are relevant, because the assumed missing value mechanisms are rather unlikely. For example in

γ_{0j2}	γ_{1j2}	$\hat{\beta}_{12}$	CI
1.0	0.2	-0.093	-0.411–0.226
5.0	1.0	-0.148	-0.471–0.176
5.0	0.2	-0.247	-0.587–0.094
0.2	1.0	0.098	-0.229–0.426
1.0	5.0	0.150	-0.194–0.493
0.2	5.0	0.206	-0.158–0.570

γ_{i12}	γ_{i22}	$\hat{\beta}_{12}$	CI
1.0	0.2	0.043	-0.281–0.366
5.0	1.0	0.054	-0.277–0.385
5.0	0.2	0.080	-0.259–0.420
0.2	1.0	-0.027	-0.341–0.287
1.0	5.0	-0.040	-0.354–0.275
0.2	5.0	-0.071	-0.388–0.246

γ_{012}	γ_{112}	γ_{022}	γ_{122}	$\hat{\beta}_{12}$	CI
0.2	1.0	1.0	0.2	-0.059	-0.376–0.259
1.0	5.0	5.0	1.0	-0.085	-0.415–0.244
0.2	5.0	5.0	0.2	-0.068	-0.428–0.291
1.0	0.2	0.2	1.0	0.121	-0.221–0.464
5.0	1.0	1.0	5.0	0.204	-0.159–0.567
5.0	0.2	0.2	5.0	0.375	-0.045–0.795

Table 8.2: Sensitivity analysis for some extreme non-MAR missing value mechanisms. Estimates of β_{12} and 95% confidence intervals.

the last row of the table we observe an estimate of 0.375 for β_{12}. For this estimate we have to assume that for unexposed controls and exposed cases a given estrogen therapy is much better documented than a non given one, but for exposed controls and unexposed cases we have to assume the opposite.

So we can conclude that in our example the estimation of the effect of exposure to radiation is not sensitive against a probable violation of the MAR assumption, whereas the estimation of the effect of the confounder is effected by such a violation.

References

Estimation under prespecified non-MAR missing value mechanisms has been discussed in the context of the analysis of categorical data by Pregibon (1977), Little (1982,1983), Nordheim (1984) and Phillips (1993). They all consider the parametrization (8.1), probably because they consider the EM algorithm as the natural tool to compute ML estimates.

Part II: Generalizations

9. General Regression Models with Missing Values in One of Two Covariates

So far we have considered the logistic regression model with two categorical covariates and missing values in one covariate. The considered techniques to handle missing values can also be applied in other regression models, at least if the covariates (and for some methods the outcome variable, too) are categorical. We will now discuss some generalizations to the case of covariates measured on an arbitrary scale, and this discussion will be done within the scope of rather general regression models. We do not consider the special case of Gaussian distributed errors, for which a lot of suggestions have been made. We refer to the excellent review of Little (1992). Note, however, that many of the methods described there depend on the assumption of a joint multivariate normal distribution of all variables.

Let be Y, X_1, X_2 random variables of arbitrary scale. The regression model relating the outcome variable Y to the covariates X_1 and X_2 is described by the conditional distribution of Y given $X_1 = x_1$ and $X_2 = x_2$ with density

$$f_\beta(y|x_1, x_2).$$

The observability of X_2 is indicated by a random variable O_2 and instead of X_2 we observe a random variable Z_2 defined analogously as in Chapter 3. The missing value mechanism is described by

$$q(y, x_1, x_2) := P(O_2 = 1|Y = y, X_1 = x_1, X_2 = x_2)$$

and the MAR assumption is $q(y, x_1, x_2) \equiv q(y, x_1)$ and the MDX assumption is $q(y, x_1, x_2) \equiv q(x_1)$.

With $g(x_2|x_1)$ denoting the density of the conditional distribution of X_2 given $X_1 = x_1$ and with $h(x_1)$ denoting the density of X_1, the joint distribution of (Y, X_1, Z_2) under the MAR assumption has the density

$$f(y, x_1, z_2) = \begin{cases} (1 - q(y, x_1)) \left[\int f_\beta(y|x_1, x_2) g(x_2|x_1) dx_2 \right] h(x_1) & \text{if } z_2 = ? \\ q(y, x_1) f_\beta(y|x_1, z_2) g(z_2|x_1) h(x_1) & \text{if } z_2 \neq ? \end{cases}$$

9.1 ML Estimation

Given a parametrization $g_\pi(x_2|x_1)$ with $\pi \in \Pi \subseteq \mathbf{R}^d$ for the conditional distributions of X_2 given $X_1 = x_1$ and assuming MAR we can estimate (β, π) by the maximum likelihood method. The contribution to the loglikelihood of a single observation (y, x_1, z_2) is

$$\ell_{ML}(\beta, \pi; y, x_1, z_2) = \begin{cases} \log \left[\int f_\beta(y|x_1, x_2) g_\pi(x_2|x_1) dx_2 \right] & \text{if } z_2 = ? \\ \log f_\beta(y|x_1, z_2) + \log g_\pi(z_2|x_1) & \text{if } z_2 \neq ? \end{cases}$$

Under regularity conditions traditional theory yields consistency, asymptotic normality and efficiency of the resulting estimates for β. Computation of the estimates can be based on a Newton-Raphson method or the EM algorithm, but the E-step may involve numerical integration (cf. Whittemore & Grosser 1986). Ibrahim & Weisberg (1992) suggest a Gaussian quadrature approximation to overcome this difficulty.

However, the crucial point is the necessity to specify a parametric family of conditional distributions with a finite number of parameters. Only if X_1 and X_2 are categorical – as considered in the main part of this book – this causes no problems, because the assumption of a multinomial distribution of X_2 given $X_1 = x_1$ for each category of X_1 yields the desired parametrization without any restriction with respect to the joint distribution of X_1 and X_2. If one or both covariates are continuous, each parametric assumption is a restriction. It is rather unlikely that we have enough knowledge about the distributions of the covariates and the relation between them to justify such a restriction, because it is one of the fundamental reasons for the popularity of regression models that they are "non-parametric" with respect to the distribution of the covariates.

9.2 Semiparametric ML Estimation

Whereas it is difficult to specify a parametric family for the conditional distributions of X_2 given $X_1 = x_1$ it seems to be rather simple to estimate them from the units with complete covariate information. With such an estimate $\hat{g}(x_2|x_1)$ estimation of β can be based on the estimated loglikelihood to which a single unit with observed values (y, x_1, z_2) contributes by

$$\hat{\ell}(\beta; y, x_1, z_2) = \begin{cases} \log\left[\int f_\beta(y|x_1, x_2)\,\hat{g}(x_2|x_1)dx_2\right] & \text{if } z_2 =? \\ \log f_\beta(y|x_1, z_2) & \text{if } z_2 \neq? \end{cases}.$$

The Pseudo Maximum Likelihood Estimation approach (Section 4.2) follows this idea for the situation of two categorical covariates. In this particular setting with a finite parametrization of $g(x_2|x_1)$ the general theory of pseudo maximum likelihood estimation enables us to show consistency and asymptotic normality of the resulting estimates for β. However, this approach suffers again from the difficulties to propose a reasonable parametrization.

Hence nonparametric estimates $\hat{g}(x_2|x_1)$ are of more interest, but suffer from the lack of a general theory establishing asymptotic properties of the estimates for β. A first step is provided by Pepe & Fleming (1991), who consider the case of a categorical covariate X_1 and a continuous covariate X_2, where $\hat{g}(x_2|x_1)$ is based on the empirical distribution of X_2 within the units with $X_1 = x_1$ and $O_2 = 1$. They prove consistency and asymptotic normality of the resulting estimates of β and suggest a method for the estimation of the asymptotic variance. To extend their approach to a continuous X_1, we can estimate $g(x_2|x_1)$ by the empirical distribution of X_2 within units with $O_2 = 1$ and X_1 in a neighborhood of x_1, for which the size depends on a bandwidth parameter. Carroll & Wand (1991) consider a similar approach in the context of a measurement error problem with validation sampling, and their techniques are probably transferable to the missing value problem.

Estimating $g(x_2|x_1)$ by the empirical distribution of X_2 within units with $O_2 = 1$ and X_1 equal or nearly equal to x_1 is based on the assumption

$$f(x_2|x_1, O_2 = 1) = f(x_2|x_1) \ .$$

This relation is implied by the MDX assumption $q(y, x_1, x_2) \equiv q(x_1)$, but not by the more general MAR assumption. However, the latter implies

$$f(x_2|x_1, y, O_2 = 1) = f(x_2|x_1, y) \ .$$

hence we can estimate $f(x_2|x_1, y)$ from the units with complete covariate information. Moreover we can estimate $f(y|x_1)$ using all units, and the estimates $\hat{f}(x_2|x_1, y)$ and $\hat{f}(y|x_1)$ can be combined to an estimate

$$\hat{f}(x_2|x_1) = \int \hat{f}(x_2|x_1, y) \, \hat{f}(y|x_1) dy \ .$$

The construction of $\tilde{\pi}^n$ in Section 4.2 follows this idea. The results of the comparison of the two types of Pseudo Maximum Likelihood Estimation in Section 5.1 suggest that this type of estimate is always preferable to the simpler estimate based on the empirical distribution of X_2 given $X_1 = x_1$ within the units with $O_2 = 1$.

As $\hat{g}(x_2|x_1)$ is a distribution with discrete support, the computation of the estimates for β involves the maximization of a likelihood, for which some units contributes with a finite mixture of distributions with known mixing fractions. This computational problem has been discussed in different settings; the EM algorithm provides a general tool for this task (cf. Aitkin & Wilson 1980, Dempster, Laird & Rubin 1977); computation within the class of generalized linear models has been discussed by Thompson & Baker (1981).

9.3 Estimation of the Score Function

In Section 4.3 we have pointed out that the Filling method can be regarded as an approach to estimate the unknown contributions to the score function. This idea can be generalized. In the complete data case the contribution of a single unit with observation (y, x_1, x_2) to the score function is

$$S^*(\beta; y, x_1, x_2) = \frac{\partial}{\partial \beta} \log f_\beta(y|x_1, x_2) \ .$$

If x_2 is unknown, the contribution to the score function is unknown, too. Now the basic property of the score function is that, evaluated at the true value of β, its expectation is equal to 0. This property is not destroyed, if we replace $S^*(\beta; y, x_1, x_2)$ by its expectation $E\left[S^*(\beta; y, x_1, X_2)\Big| Y = y, X_1 = x_1, O_2 = 0\right]$ if X_2 is unobserved, and the MAR assumption allows to omit the condition $O_2 = 0$. If both X_1 and Y are categorical variables it is straightforward to estimate this expectation by the average of the values $S^*(y_r, x_{1r}, x_{2r})$ of the units with $y_r = y$ and $x_{1r} = x_1$ and observed X_2. Reilly (1991) and Reilly & Pepe (1993a) call this approach the "Mean Score Method"; they show consistency and asymptotic normality of the resulting estimates for β and give an explicit representation of the asymptotic variance. The estimated score function can then be expressed as

$$n\hat{S}^{*n}(\beta) = \sum_{\substack{r \\ O_{2r}=1}} S^*(\beta; y_r, x_{1r}, x_{2r}) + \sum_{\substack{r \\ O_{2r}=0}} \frac{\sum_{r' \text{ with } O_{2r'}=1, y_{r'}=y_r, x_{1r'}=x_{1r}} S^*(\beta; y_{r'}, x_{1r'}, x_{2r'})}{\#\{r'|O_{2r'} = 1, y_{r'} = y_r, x_{1r'} = x_{1r}\}}$$

$$= \sum_{\substack{r \\ O_{2r}=1}} S^*(\beta; y_r, x_{1r}, z_{2r}) \left(1 + \frac{\#\{r'|O_{2r'} = 0, y_{r'} = y_r, x_{1r'} = x_{1r}\}}{\#\{r'|O_{2r'} = 1, y_{r'} = y_r, x_{1r'} = x_{1r}\}} \right)$$

$$= \sum_{\substack{r \\ O_{2r}=1}} \frac{S^*(\beta; y_r, x_{1r}, z_{2r})}{\hat{q}(y_r, x_{1r})} \quad \text{with } \hat{q}(y, x_1) := \frac{\#\{r|O_{2r} = 1, y_r = y, x_{1r} = x_1\}}{\#\{r|y_r = y, x_{1r} = x_1\}},$$

i.e., the contribution of a unit with complete covariate information is weighted reciprocally to an estimate of the unit's observation probability. Hence Filling is a special case of the Mean Score Method with categorical X_2.

The extension to continuous Y and/or X_1 has not yet been considered, although the first basic step is rather simple: The estimation of $E[S^*(\beta; y, x_1, X_2)|Y = y, X_1 = x_1]$ is the classical problem of non-parametric regression. Following the general approach of Stone (1977) on nonparametric regression, we have weight functions $(w_r(x, y))_{r, O_r=1}$, such that

$$\hat{s}(\beta; x, y) := \sum_{\substack{r \\ O_r=1}} w_r(x, y) \cdot S^*(\beta; y_r, x_{1r}, x_{2r})$$

is a consistent estimate for $E[S^*(\beta; y, x_1, X_2)|Y = y, X_1 = x_1, O = 1]$, and the MAR assumption allows to omit $O = 1$. The estimated score function is now

$$n\hat{S}^{*n}(\beta) = \sum_{\substack{r \\ O_{2r}=1}} S^*(\beta; y_r, x_{1r}, x_{2r}) + \sum_{\substack{s \\ O_{2s}=0}} \hat{s}(\beta; x_s, y_s)$$

$$= \sum_{\substack{r \\ O_{2r}=1}} S^*(\beta; y_r, x_{1r}, x_{2r}) + \sum_{\substack{s \\ O_{2s}=0}} \sum_{\substack{r \\ O_{2r}=1}} w_r(x_s, y_s) S^*(\beta; y_r, x_{1r}, x_{2r})$$

$$= \sum_{\substack{r \\ O_{2r}=1}} S^*(\beta; y_r, x_{1r}, x_{2r}) v_r^n \quad \text{with } v_r^n := 1 + \sum_{\substack{s \\ O_{2s}=0}} w_r(x_s, y_s).$$

Again, the estimated score function is a weighted sum of the contributions of the completely observed units. This allows again the use of standard software to compute the estimates. The weights v_r^n can be regarded as estimates for $q(y_r, x_{1r})^{-1}$. It remains to show consistency and asymptotic normality of the resulting estimate for β and to find a procedure to estimate its variance. This task has not yet been solved. Furthermore the use of nearest neighbour techniques as well as the use of kernel estimates to construct the weight functions $(w_r(x, y))_{r, O_r=1}$ requires the use of an appropriate distance measure on the space where Y_1 and X_1 are measured, and guidelines for the appropriate choice of bandwidth parameters are desired.

The relation between ML Estimation and Filling can also be extended to this general procedure. The contribution of a single unit with observation $(y, x_1, ?)$ to the score function of ML Estimation can be expressed as

$$E_{\beta, \pi} \left[S^*(\beta; y, x_1, X_2) \middle| Y = y, X_1 = x_1 \right]$$

(cf. Tanner 1991, p.37), hence estimating the expectation non-parametrically neglects the dependence on the regression parameter. The comparison between ML Estimation and Filling by means of asymptotic relative efficiency (Section 5.2) may suggest that this neglection is irrelevant under the MCAR assumption.

An alternative approach of generalization may directly try to estimate the function $q(y, x_1)^{-1}$ in order to obtain weights for the contributions of the completely observed units. However, this appealing idea seems to be misleading. The best estimate for $q(y, x_1)^{-1}$ is $q(y, x_1)^{-1}$ itself, but then under the MCAR assumption we have to weight each contribution by a constant and we obtain the complete case estimates. Hence under the MCAR assumption no gain in efficiency is possible.

One attractive aspect of the approach to estimate the unknown contributions to the score function is its applicability to all methods, where estimation equations are formed by adding contributions of each unit. Hence it is not restricted to regression models fully specifying the conditional distributions.

9.4 Complete Case Analysis

The Complete Case Analysis is based on the implicit assumption

$$f_\beta(y|x_1, x_2, O_2 = 1) = f_\beta(y|x_1, x_2) .$$

A sufficient condition for the validity of this assumption is

$$q(y, x_1, x_2) \equiv q(x_1, x_2) . \tag{9.1}$$

This condition is quite different from the MAR assumption. It requires that there is no relation between the outcome variable and the occurrence of missing values in X_2, which cannot be explained by X_1 and X_2. With respect to this point, it is stronger than the MAR assumption. However, it allows that the occurrence of missing values in X_2 depends on the covariates, and especially on X_2 itself. With respect to this point, it is contrary to the MAR assumption. This robustness against violations of the MAR assumption is a useful property in many applications, and it has to be weighted against a potentially unnecessary waste of information. We will discuss this in the light of some examples in Chapter 12.

The sufficiency of condition (9.1) can easily be verified, because

$$f_\beta(y|x_1, x_2, O_2 = 1) = \frac{q(y, x_1, x_2) \cdot f_\beta(y|x_1, x_2)}{\int q(y, x_1, x_2) \cdot f_\beta(y|x_1, x_2) \, dy} .$$

It is also intuitively clear, because it requires that the selection of units available in the Complete Case Analysis depends only on the covariate values, i.e., we change only the distribution of the covariates in the analysed population without changing the regression model.

However, it is well-known that the distribution of the covariates has a strong impact on the precision of the regression parameter estimates. For example let X_2 be the average daily alcohol consumption of a unit. If data for this variable is based on a questionnaire then $q(x_1, x_2)$ may increase rapidly with increasing x_2, such that only very few units with a high value of x_2 remain in the population available for the Complete Case Analysis, and hence the estimate $\hat{\beta}_2$ of the influence of x_2 will show a large standard deviation. Keeping the global observation rate q_A fixed, the precision would increase, if $q(x_1, x_2)$ does not depend on x_2. Additionally we must be aware that the robustness property of the Complete Case Analysis strongly depends on the assumption that the model $f_\beta(y|x_1, x_2)$ is correctly specified. If in the example above there exists an interaction between x_1 and x_2 which is not included in the model, then the Complete Case Analysis tends to estimate the effect of x_1 for low level drinkers. Without missing values, we would instead estimate a weighted average of the effect of X_1 for low and high level drinkers. Moreover, we may often take into account the existence of a latent variable like "positive attitude to clinical medicine" or "positive attitude to social or economical questionnaires", which may have some impact on the occurrence of missing values. This latent variable may be associated with the outcome variable, too, or there may be an interaction between this latent variable and some covariates, which may be the cause of misleading results from the Complete Case Analysis.

It should be mentioned that there may be weaker conditions than (9.1) to assure consistency of the estimates of a Complete Case Analysis, especially if we only want to estimate certain components of β. For example if we consider the logistic model

$$f_\beta(y|x_1, x_2) = \Lambda(\beta_0 + \beta_1 x_1 + \beta_2 x_2)^y (1 - \Lambda(\beta_0 + \beta_1 x_1 + \beta_2 x_2))^{1-y}$$

then it suffices that $q(y, x_1, x_2)$ can be decomposed as

$$q(y, x_1, x_2) = q_1(y) \cdot q_2(x_1, x_2)$$

in order to assure consistent estimation of β_1 and β_2. This follows from

$$f_\beta(y|x_1, x_2, O_2 = 1) = \frac{q_1(y) \cdot f_\beta(y|x_1, x_2)}{\int q_1(y) \cdot f_\beta(y|x_1, x_2)\, dy} = f_{\tilde\beta}(y|x_1, x_2)$$

with $\tilde\beta_0 = \log \dfrac{q_1(1)}{q_1(0)} + \beta_0$, $\tilde\beta_1 = \beta_1$, and $\tilde\beta_2 = \beta_2$,

This is just the argument justifying the use of logistic regression models in the analysis of case-control studies, cf. Breslow & Day (1980), p. 203.

9.5 Mean Imputation and Additional Category

At the present state it seems to be difficult to give a general judgement about conditional mean imputation, because its properties seem to depend on the particular regression model. To illustrate this, let us assume that the MDX assumption is valid. Then we have

$$f_\beta(y|x_1, z_2) = \begin{cases} f_\beta(y|x_1, z_2) & \text{if } z_2 \neq ? \\ \int f_\beta(y|x_1, x_2)\, g(x_2|x_1)\, dx_2 & \text{if } z_2 = ? \end{cases}.$$

The implicit modeling of conditional mean imputation coincides for $z_2 \neq ?$, but otherwise we have

$$f_\beta(y|x_1, ?) = f_\beta\left(y|x_1, E(X_2|X_1 = x_1)\right).$$

To evaluate this difference, we consider the modeled conditional expectations of Y. With

$\mu_\beta(x_1, x_2) := E_\beta[Y|X_1 = x_1, X_2 = x_2]$ we have

$$\tilde{\mu}_\beta(y, x_1) := E_\beta[Y|X_1 = x_1, Z_2 =?] = \int \mu_\beta(x_1, x_2) \cdot f(x_2|x_1)\, dx_1$$

whereas Conditional Mean Imputation assumes

$$\tilde{\mu}_\beta(x_1, ?) = \tilde{\tilde{\mu}}_\beta(x_1, ?)$$

with $\qquad \tilde{\tilde{\mu}}_\beta(x_1, ?) := \mu_\beta \left(x_1, \int x_2 f(x_2|x_1)\, dx_2 \right) .$

Equality holds, if $\mu(x_1, x_2)$ is linear in its second argument, especially if

$$\mu_\beta(x_1, x_2) = \beta_0 + \beta_1 x_1 + \beta_2 x_2 \tag{9.2}$$

Hence imputation of exact conditional expectations would result in a correct specification of the expectation, and only the type of the distribution (and hence the variance) is misspecified. Hence it is not surprising that under very general conditions Conditional Mean Imputation results in consistent estimates for the regression parameters, if (9.2) holds (Gill 1986), whereas estimates of the variance are mostly invalid. Also many other papers about Mean Imputation start with the assumption (9.2) (e.g. Hill & Ziemer 1983, Nijman & Palm 1988). For many regression models including the logistic one (9.2) is not satisfied, and hence we have asymptotically biased estimates.

The second point is the specification of the variance. Let us consider generalized linear models where

$$Var(Y|X_1 = x_1, X_2 = x_2) = \sigma^2 \cdot V(\mu_\beta(x_1, x_2)) .$$

Then

$$Var(Y|X_1 = x_1, Z_2 =?) = \sigma^2 \cdot \int V(\mu_\beta(x_1, x_2)) f(x_2|x_1)\, dx_2$$

$$+ \int (\mu_\beta(x_1, x_2))^2 f(x_2|x_1)\, dx_2 - \left(\int \mu_\beta(x_1, x_2) f(x_2|x_1)\, dx_2 \right)^2$$

Conditional Mean Imputation assumes incorrectly

$$Var(Y|X_1 = x_1, Z_2 =?) = \sigma^2 \cdot V\left(\tilde{\mu}_\beta(x_1, ?) \right) .$$

For binary outcome variables the difference is small, because $\sigma^2 = 1$ and

$$Var(Y|X_1 = x_1, Z_2 =?) = V(\tilde{\mu}_\beta(x_1, ?)) ,$$

hence the misspecification of the variance is just a function of the misspecification of the expectation. For continuous outcome variables the difference may be much larger, which may have some impact on the validity of variance estimation, cf. Gill (1986). Hence the results of our simulation study in Section 6.3 cannot be directly generalized for other regression models with respect to the validity of confidence intervals. Within the theory of least squares estimation several suggestions to weight down observations with missing values have been made, cf. Dagenais (1973), Beale & Little (1975) and again Gill (1986).

So far we have assumed that we can compute $E(X_2|X_1 = x_1)$ directly. Mean imputation requires to estimate these quantities. It would be too restrictive in most applications to assume that $E(X_2|X_1 = x_1)$ is linear in x_1, hence this step requires methods of nonparametric regression. As these estimates are less efficient than parametric estimates, the neglection of their variance in determining the variance of $\hat{\beta}$ may have a stronger impact on the validity of confidence intervals, too.

The imputation of unconditional means, i.e. of estimates for EX_2, seems to be only justified if X_1 and X_2 are independent. Under this assumption it may also be justified to regard missing values as an additional category. If X_2 is continuous, this means that we set X_2 to 0 if $Z_2 =?$ and add an indication variable for missingness in the model. The corresponding parameter β_3 replaces EX_2, if we compare this approach to unconditional mean imputation.

In general, Unconditional Mean Imputation and Additional Category seem to be no recommendable approaches to handle missing values even if the MAR assumption is valid. However, Additional Category may be a good tool if the MAR assumption is totally violated, if for example X_2 is unobservable for only one category of X_2, or if missingness is highly correlated with the outcome variable. For instance Commenges et al. (1992) report of a study containing several psychological tests to improve diagnosis of dementia for screening purposes. They found that missing values for Benton's Visual Retention Test or Isaac's Set Test have a high predictive value. This is not surprising, because these missing values are probably due to the total disability of the subjects to understand the tests.

9.6 The Cox Proportional Hazards Model

For the analysis of (censored) failure times the Cox proportional hazards model plays a similar role as the logistic regression model for the analysis of binary data. However, the proportional hazards model does not fit into the framework of the preceding sections, because the distribution of the failure times is specified only in part. Hence the concepts considered need some adjustments.

For a random variable T with density $f(t)$ the hazard function $\lambda(t)$ is defined as

$$\lambda(t) := \frac{f(t)}{P(T \geq t)} \ .$$

In the general setting of failure time intensity models the hazard function of the failure time of a unit with covariate values $X_1 = x_1$ and $X_2 = x_2$ is decomposed as

$$\lambda(t|x_1, x_2) = \lambda_0(t) \cdot r(\beta; x_1, x_2, t) \ .$$

The baseline hazard function $\lambda_0(t)$ is unspecified, and $r(\beta; x_1, x_2, t)$ is a known function with unknown parameter β. If $r(\beta; x_1, x_2, t)$ is independent of t, we have a proportional hazards model; i.e., the ratio of the hazard functions of two different units is constant over time. In the Cox model (Cox, 1972) we have $r(\beta; x_1, x_2, t) = \exp(\beta_1 x_1 + \beta_2 x_2)$. Here with X_2 fixed a change of 1 on the scale of X_1 results in a relative risk of $\exp(\beta_1)$ to fail at time t given to be at risk at time t for any t. Given for n units the observed times $(Y_i)_{i=1,\dots,n}$, censoring indicators $(\delta_i)_{i=1,\dots,n}$ and covariate values $(X_{1i}, X_{2i})_{i=1,\dots,n}$, statistical inference is based on the partial likelihood

$$PL(\beta) = \prod_{\substack{i=1 \\ \delta_i=0}}^{n} \frac{r(\beta; X_{1i}, X_{2i}, Y_i)}{\sum_{j \in R(T_i)} r(\beta, X_{1j}, X_{2j}, Y_j)}$$

where $R(t) := \{j | Y_j \geq t\}$ is the set of units to be at risk at time t. A maximum partial likelihood estimate for β can now be achieved by solving the equations $\frac{\partial}{\partial \beta} \log PL(\beta) = 0$.

In the presence of missing values we observe the covariate Z_2 instead of X_2. Under the MDX assumption the hazard function of the conditional distribution of T given $X_1 = x_1$ and $Z_2 = z_2$ is

$$\lambda(t|x_1, z_2) = \begin{cases} \lambda(t|x_1, z_2) & \text{if } z_2 \neq ? \\ \frac{\int f(t|x_1, x_2) \cdot f(x_2|x_1)\, dx_2}{P(T \geq t|X_1 = x_1)} & \text{if } z_2 = ? \end{cases}$$

For $z_2 = ?$ we have further

$$\lambda(t|x_1, ?)$$

$$= \frac{\int \lambda(t|x_1, x_2) \cdot P(T \geq t|X_1 = x_1, X_2 = x_2) \cdot f(x_2|x_1)\, dx_2}{P(T \geq t|X_1 = x_1)}$$

$$= \lambda_0(t) \cdot \int r(\beta; x_1, x_2, t) \cdot f(x_2|T \geq t, X_1 = x_1)\, dx_2$$

$$= \lambda_0(t) \cdot \tilde{r}(\beta; x_1, t)$$

with $\tilde{r}(\beta; x_1, t) := E[r(\beta; x_1, X_2, t)|T \geq t, X_1 = x_1]$,

cf. Prentice (1982). Hence even if we start with a proportional hazards model, missing values in the covariates result in non-proportional hazards. This makes it evident that strategies like Additional Category or Mean Imputation are potentially dangerous here, because the final analysis is based on the assumption of proportional hazards.

For a more sophisticated approach we have to solve the problem that $\tilde{r}(\beta; x_1, t)$ is unknown, because it depends on the conditional distribution of X_2 given X_1 and on the conditional distribution of T. In analogy to semiparametric ML estimation one can try to estimate $\tilde{r}(\beta; x_1, t)$ from the data, such that estimation of β can be based on an estimated partial likelihood. For a categorical X_1 this approach has been considered in detail by Zhou & Pepe (1993). The estimate for $\tilde{r}(\beta; x_1, t)$ is then

$$\left(\sum_{\substack{i \\ Y_i \geq t, X_{1i} = x_1, O_{2i} = 1}} r(\beta; x_1, X_{2i}, t) \right) \Big/ \#\{i | Y_i \geq t, X_{1i} = x_1, O_{2i} = 1\}$$

which is based on censored as well as on uncensored units.

The approach to estimate the contribution to the score function for units with missing values is faced with the following difficulty. The contribution of a unit with uncensored failure time

Y and covariate values X_1 and X_2 is given by

$$\frac{\frac{\partial}{\partial \beta} r(\beta; X_1, X_2, Y)}{r(\beta; X_1, X_2, Y)} - \frac{\sum_{j \in R(t)} \frac{\partial}{\partial \beta} r(\beta; X_{1j}, X_{2j}, Y)}{\sum_{j \in R(t)} r(\beta; X_{1j}, X_{2j}, Y)} .$$

It depends on all covariate values of the units which are at risk at time Y. Hence each missing value in X_2 causes the contribution to the score function to be unknown for all units with a smaller observation time. To overcome this difficulty it is allowed under the MDX assumption to restrict the denominator of the partial likelihood to complete cases. Then it is possible to estimate the contributions of units with a missing value by non-parametric regression. Pugh et al. (1993) present a similar approach; the contributions to the score function of the complete data case are weighted reciprocally to estimated observation probabilities. The latter are based on fitting a logistic regression model to the response indicator. However, this approach is subject to the criticism mentioned at the end of Section 9.3, too. Nevertheless, the approach is valuable in the special setting of case-cohort designs where missing rates depend on censoring, such that a Complete Case Analysis yields biased estimates. If the observation probabilities depend neither on the failure time nor on the censoring indicator, Complete Case Analysis yields consistent estimates.

10. Generalizations for More Than two Covariates

We now consider the case, where we have not 2, but $p > 2$ covariates $X_1, \ldots, X_p$. We do not consider Mean/Probability Imputation and Additional Category, because the basic criticism presented in Chapter 4 and 9 of course remains valid. Also Complete Case Analysis is not considered in detail, but we should mention that the robustness against violations of the MAR assumption remains valid of course, too. Thus we restrict our attention in this chapter to ML Estimation, Semiparametric ML Estimation, and Estimation of the Score Function.

10.1 One Covariate with Missing Values

In this Section we assume that $X_1, \ldots, X_{p-1}$ are completely observed, and that only X_p may be affected by missing values. The conceptual ideas of ML Estimation, Semiparametric ML Estimation, and Estimation of the Score Function need not be changed in this situation. However, due to the increasing number of dimensions a lot of problems in the technical implementation of the basic concepts appear.

ML Estimation

The basic difficulty of specifying a parametric family of the conditional distributions of X_p given $X_1, \ldots, X_{p-1}$ remains. Even if all covariates are categorical, it may now be necessary to set up restrictions on the joint distribution of the covariates, because a saturated model may result in too many nuisance parameters. For example if $p = 6$ and all covariates have three categories, this approach results in 486 nuisance parameters in contrast to 13 remaining parameters of interest. Log-linear models with restrictions on the order of interaction are then a feasible alternative, cf. Chapter 12. If additionally X_p is binary this results in a linear logistic model for the conditional distribution, which may also be used if some of the covariates $X_1, \ldots, X_{p-1}$ are continuous.

Semiparametric ML Estimation

Here the basic task is to find non-parametric estimates for the conditional distributions of X_p given $X_1, \ldots, X_{p-1}$. Hence we have to find an appropriate distance measure on the space where $X_1, \ldots, X_{p-1}$ is measured, which is especially difficult if the variables are measured on different scales.

Estimation of the Score Function

Here we have to conduct a non-parametric regression of $S_\beta(Y, X_1, \ldots, X_{p-1}, X_p)$ on $Y, X_1, \ldots, X_{p-1}$. Hence we need an appropriate distance measure on the space where $Y, X_1, \ldots, X_{p-1}$ is measured. Besides the increase of dimension there exists a further remarkable difference between this approach and (semiparametric) ML estimation. We know that in randomized experiments one or several covariates are independent of the remaining covariates. This knowledge leads to a decrease of the dimension of the space to be considered in (semiparametric) ML estimation. This simplification does not appear in the estimation of the score function.

10.2 Missing Values in More Than one Covariate

Compared to the preceding section we have two additional difficulties. First for (semiparametric) ML estimation we now have to consider multivariate instead of univariate distributions. Second the idea of the semiparametric approaches to estimate the necessary quantities from the units with complete covariate information is obviously inefficient. E.g. if we want to estimate the conditional distribution of X_1 and X_2 given $X_3, \ldots, X_p$, information is available from units where only X_1 or only X_2 is missing, but this is neglected using only units with complete covariate information. In the extreme case where we have a missing value in at least one covariate for all units, there remain no units to be used.

ML Estimation

If all covariates are affected by missing values, we have to specify the joint distribution of all covariates, otherwise it may be enough to specify the conditional distribution of the covariates affected by missing values given the covariates not affected by missing values. It is important to note that in the implementation of ML estimation it is additionally necessary to compute marginal distributions of the multivariate conditional distributions. If for example X_1, X_2 and X_3 are affected by missing values and a family $f_\theta(x_1, x_2, x_3 | x_4, \ldots, x_p)$ is specified, a unit with a missing value only in X_1 and X_2 requires for the computation of the log-likelihood an expression for $\int \int f_\theta(x_1, x_2, x_3 | x_4, \ldots, x_p)\, dx_1\, dx_2$. If all covariates are categorical, log-linear models provide a useful framework.

Semiparametric ML Estimation

Here it is the basic task to find for any occurring missing pattern $\mathcal{M} \subseteq \{1, \ldots, p\}$ an appropriate non-parametric estimate for the conditional distribution of $(X_j)_{j \in \mathcal{M}}$ given $(X_j)_{j \in \{1, \ldots, p\} \setminus \mathcal{M}}$, based on the units with complete covariate information. A straightforward idea to improve the efficiency is the following sequential procedure. We first estimate the conditional distributions for units with one missing value. Then in estimating the conditional distributions for units with two missing values units with one missing value can be used, too, if we represent them by a distribution, not by a single value, and so on. Additionally one may start with estimating the conditional distribution for units with a missing value only in the first covariate and may use these estimates already in the estimation of conditional distributions for units with missing values in the second covariate. However, the final estimates now depend on the sequence of the covariates, and an optimal procedure seems to require an iterative procedure.

Estimation of the Score Function

Here it is the basic task to conduct for any missing pattern $\mathcal{M}$ a non-parametric regression of $S_\beta(Y, X_1, \ldots, X_p)$ on $Y, (X_j)_{j \in \{1, \ldots, p\} \setminus \mathcal{M}}$, based on the observations with complete covariate information. Note, that here the dimensionality of the outcome variable of the regression problem does not increase with the number of covariates affected by missing values. A sequential procedure to improve these estimates is straightforward. Alternatively, if all variables are categorical, we can use the ML estimates of the cell probabilities under a multinomial model, extending the Filling method. Computation of these ML estimates requires an iterative method, if the missing pattern is not monotone (cf. Little & Rubin (1987), p. 181).

Baker, Rosenberger & Dersimonian (1992) consider assumptions slightly different from MAR which allow explicit representations of efficient estimates of the cell probabilities.

11. Missing Values and Subsampling

A special type of missing values in the covariates is due to sampling schemes, where some covariates are measured only for a subsample. As this subsample is planned in advance, the missing value mechanism satisfies the MAR assumption. We consider in this chapter the application of ML estimation, semiparametric ML estimation and estimation of the score function in this setting. Modifications of these approaches are necessary, if the subsample is a validation sample with precise measurements of a covariate, for which a surrogate covariate is measured for all subjects. Finally we consider subsampling of the nonresponders and the sampling of additional variables to avoid a violation of the MAR assumption.

11.1 Two Stage Designs

If the collection of some variables is very expensive, one may decide in advance to collect these variables only for a subset of all units, whereas other variables are collected for all units. In the epidemiological literature this sampling procedure is called a two stage design; however, in the literature on survey sampling the terms *double sampling* or *two phase sampling* are preferred (Cochran 1977, chapter 12). As the decision on the occurrence of missing values is made in advance, the missing value mechanism satisfies the MAR assumption. Indeed, many suggestions to analyze data from a two stage design are related to methods considered in this book. The first suggestion of White (1982) is a complete case analysis with a correction for the bias. This correction is necessary, as she considers case control studies with a rare exposure and suggests to sample in the second stage more frequently from the exposed than from the unexposed. Additionally she considers sampling rates depending on the case control status, such that we have a biased estimate of the risk associated with exposure (cf. Section 4.4 and Vach & Blettner 1991). In the more recent literature we can find suggestions for pseudo maximum likelihood estimation (Breslow & Cain 1988, Wild 1991, Zhao & Lipsitz 1992) as well as suggestions to estimate the score function (Flanders & Greenland 1991, Wild 1991, Zhao & Lipsitz 1992). These approaches are sometimes a little bit different from those in this book, as they consider the second stage as a part of the retrospective sampling of a case control study with fixed sampling fractions. The methods of this book require that for each unit an independent, random decision to be sampled or not is made. It remains to investigate, whether the approach to analyze retrospective studies by prospective logistic regression models remains always valid in the presence of missing values by design.

11.2 Surrogate Covariates and Validation Sampling

If the precise measurement of a covariate is expensive, but collection of a surrogate is cheap, one may decide to collect the surrogate covariate for all units, but to measure the covariate precisely only for a subsample in order to estimate the relation between the covariate and its surrogate. This type of validation sampling is hoped to be a solution to the measurement error and misclassification problems in clinical and epidemiological studies (cf. Byar & Gail, 1989). We consider the situation with one outcome variable Y, one covariate X_1 observable for all units and one surrogate S_2 for the covariate X_2. S_2 is observable for all units, but the precise measurement Z_2 of X_2 is only available in the validation sample, i.e., $Z_2 = ?$ for the units not in the validation sample. As the validation sample is planned in advance, [10†] we can assume

$$q(y, x_1, x_2, s_2) \equiv q(y, x_1, s_2) \tag{11.1}$$

with $q(y, x_1, x_2, s_2) := P(Z_2 = ?|Y = y, X_1 = x_1, X_2 = x_2, S_2 = s_2)$

i.e. the MAR assumption holds. Compared to the situation considered in Chapter 9, we have the additional variable S_2, but this variable is not a covariate in our regression model. Excluding additionally a dependence of the validation sample fractions on the outcome variable, i.e. assuming $q(y, x_1, s_2) \equiv q(x_1, s_2)$, we find for the conditional distribution of Y given X_1, S_2 and Z_2

$$f(y|x_1, s_2, z_2) = \begin{cases} \int f_\beta(y|x_1, x_2) \cdot g(x_2|s_2, x_1)\,dx_2 & \text{if } z_2 = ? \\ f_\beta(y|x_1, z_2) \cdot g(z_2|s_2, x_1) & \text{if } z_2 \neq ? \end{cases} \tag{11.2}$$

where $g(x_2|s_2, x_1)$ is the density of the conditional distribution of X_2 given $S_2 = s_2$ and $X_1 = x_1$. Specifying a parametric family for g, we can conduct a ML estimation. Alternatively we may estimate g from the validation sample and receive a pseudo (or semiparametric) ML estimate by maximizing the estimated likelihood analogously to Section 9.2. This approach is considered by Pepe & Fleming (1991) for categorical X_1 and S_2, by Carroll & Wand (1991) for a simple continuous surrogate variable without additional covariates, and by Schill et al. (1993) for a likelihood based on a retrospective sampling scheme.

If the validation sample fractions depend on the outcome variable, a likelihood based approach can be based on the joint distribution of Y, X_1, S_2 and Z_2. However it is now essential whether the relation between the true covariate X_2 and the surrogate variable S_2 depends on Y or not. More precisely, we have to distinguish the cases

$$f(s_2|y, x_1, x_2) \equiv f(s_2|x_1, x_2) \tag{11.3}$$

and

$$f(s_2|y, x_1, x_2) \text{ depends on } y\ . \tag{11.4}$$

This corresponds to the distinction between *non-differential* and *differential* measurement error, cf. Willett (1989) and Walker & Lanes (1991). Now if we assume (11.3) and (11.1) we find for the joint distribution

$$f(y, x_1, s_2, z_2) \propto \begin{cases} \int f_\beta(y|x_1, x_2) \cdot g(x_2|s_2, x_1)\,dx_2 & \text{if } z_2 = ? \\ f_\beta(y|x_1, z_2) \cdot g(z_2|s_2, x_1) & \text{if } z_2 \neq ? \end{cases}$$

such that we can proceed as above. If we have to assume (11.4), we find for the joint distribution under (11.1)

[10†] We assume here and in the following that the validation sample is planned only based on the knowledge of the variables Y, X_1 and S_2. If other variables additionally influence the sampling fractions, and these variables are correlated with X_2, (11.1) may be violated.

$$f(y, x_1, s_2, z_2) \propto \begin{cases} \int h(s_2|y, x_1, x_2) \cdot f_\beta(y|x_1, x_2) \cdot g(x_2|x_1)\, dx_2 & \text{if } z_2 =? \\ h(s_2|y, x_1, z_2) \cdot f_\beta(y|x_1, z_2) \cdot g(z_2|x_1) & \text{if } z_2 \neq? \end{cases} \qquad (11.5)$$

where $g(x_2|x_1)$ denotes the density of the conditional distribution of X_2 given $X_1 = x_1$ and $h(s_2|y, x_1, x_2)$ denotes the density of the conditional distribution of S_2 given $Y = y$, $X_1 = x_1$ and $X_2 = x_2$. ML estimation requires now a parametrization of g and h, whereas semiparametric ML estimation can be based on estimates for g and/or h based on the validation sample. Naive estimates for h are only valid, if the validation sample probabilities $q(y, x_1, s_2)$ do not depend on s_2, otherwise appropriate adjustments are necessary.

The situation where the missing rates do not depend on the outcome variable and we have a differential measurement error calls for further attention. Here we can use both approaches, but there is an argument that estimation based on (11.5) is preferable. If the measurement error is differential, the conditional distribution of X_2 given X_1 and S_2 is a mixture of possibly very different distributions and has hence a large variance, such that units out of the validation sample are regarded as little informative in the likelihood based on (11.2). Estimation based on (11.5) seems to avoid this.

An alternative to likelihood based approaches is the estimation of the score function. Analogously to Section 9.3 we have to replace for a unit out of the validation sample the unknown contribution $S_\beta^*(y, x_1, x_2)$ to the score function by its expectation given the observed variables, i.e. by

$$E\left[S_\beta^*(y, x_1, X_2)|Y = y, X_1 = x_1, O_2 = 0, S_2 = s_2 \right].$$

With appropriate weight functions $(w_r(y, x_1, s_2)_{r,O_{2r}=1})$ the estimate

$$\hat{s}(\beta; y, x_1, s_2) := \sum_{\substack{r \\ O_{2r}=1}} w_r(y, x_1, s_2) \cdot S^*(\beta; y_r, x_{1r}, x_{2r})$$

is consistent for $E\left[S^*(\beta; y, x_1, X_2)|Y = y, X_1 = x_1, S_2 = s_2, O_2 = 1\right]$, and the assumption (11.1) allows to omit $O_2 = 1$. For the case that Y, X_1 and S_2 are categorical, this approach is examined in detail by Reilly (1991) and Reilly & Pepe (1993a).

11.3 Subsampling of the Nonresponders

Subsampling can be also used to investigate the missing value mechanism if the MAR assumption is in doubt. In a second stage of data collection a new attempt is started to gather information for a subsample of units with missing values in the first stage. This procedure is well known in survey sampling (e.g. Hansen & Hurwitz 1946, Rao 1983), but also used in medical studies (e.g. Toutenburg & Walther 1992). The crucial point is to find a strategy to attain complete information at the second stage. If this is possible, statistical inference of the regression parameters is possible, too.

We consider the situation, where the outcome variable Y and the first covariate X_1 is always observable, whereas instead of the second covariate X_2 we observe Z_2 in the first stage and Z_2' in the second stage, such that

$$Z_2' = \begin{cases} X_2 & \text{if the unit is a member of the subsample of the second stage} \\ ? & \text{otherwise} \end{cases}$$

As the subsample of the second stage includes only units with a missing value in the first stage, we have $Z_2 \neq ? \Rightarrow Z_2' =?$. We have to distinguish the observation probabilities

$$q(y, x_1, x_2) = P(Z_2 \neq ?|Y = y, X_1 = x_1, X_2 = x_2)$$

and

$$q'(y, x_1, x_2) = P(Z_2' \neq ?|Y = y, X_1 = x_1, X_2 = x_2, Z_2 =?) \ .$$

The basic assumption is

$$q'(y, x_1, x_2) \equiv q'(y, x_1)$$

which is of course satisfied, if in the second stage all units of the subsample respond. Under this assumption a likelihood based approach can be based on the joint distribution of Y, X_1, Z_2 and Z_2'. We find (with the notation of Chapter 9)

$$f(y, x_1, z_2, z_2') \propto \begin{cases} q(y, x_1, z_2) \cdot f_\beta(y|x_1, z_2) \cdot g(z_2|x_1) & \text{if } z_2 \neq? \\ (1 - q(y, x_1, z_2')) \cdot f_\beta(y|x_1, z_2') \cdot g(z_2'|x_1) & \text{if } z_2 \neq? \text{ and } z_2' \neq? \\ \int (1 - q(y, x_1, x_2)) \cdot f_\beta(y|x_1, x_2) \cdot g(x_2|x_1) \, dx_2 & \text{if } z_2 =? \text{ and } z_2' =? \end{cases}$$

Specifying parametric families for q and g estimation by the ML principle is possible. Alternatively we can estimate q and/or g in a nonparametric manner and maximize the estimated likelihood. In the construction of these estimates one has to consider the subsampling fractions $q'(y, x_1)$ in an appropriate manner. Alternative estimation of the regression parameters can be based on an estimated score function. Analogously to Section 9.3 we have now to base the nonparametric regression estimates on the subsample of the nonresponders.

11.4 (Sub-)Sampling of additional variables

In some situations a violation of the MAR assumption is not caused by a direct dependency of the observability on the true value, but by a joint dependence of the variable and its observability on a third variable. For example in a study collecting data on a covariate like diet one may observe that the observation rates depend on education and age. Hence even if diet and its observability are independent given education and age, the MAR assumption is violated in the analysis of a regression model, where diet is a covariate, but education and/or age are omitted. Hence it may be wise to consider additional variables in the analysis without using them as covariates. For the conditional distribution for such a variable X_3 we can assume that

$$f(x_3|y, x_1, x_2) \equiv f(x_3|x_1, x_2) \ .$$

Then estimation can be based on

$$f(y, x_1, z_2, x_3) \propto \begin{cases} f_\beta(y|x_1, z_2) \cdot h(z_2|x_1, x_3) & \text{if } z_2 \neq ? \\ \int f_\beta(y|x_1, x_2) \cdot h(x_2|x_1, x_3) \, dx_2 & \text{if } z_2 = ? \end{cases},$$

where the conditional distribution $h(x_2|x_1, x_3)$ is either to be parametrized or to be estimated in a nonparametric manner.

However, to be realistic, X_3 may be also affected by missing values or we may decide in advance to collect data on X_3 only for a subsample of all units. So we observe instead of X_3 the random variable Z_3 and the observability indicator O_3. For the second part of the missing value mechanism given by

$$P(O_3|Y = y, X_1 = x_1, X_2 = x_2, O_2 = o_2, X_3 = x_3) =: q'(y, x_1, x_2, o_2, x_3)$$

we have now to assume that there is no dependence on x_2 and x_3. We allow a dependence on the observability of X_2, which is important, because the occurrence of missing values in different variables is seldomly independent. So we start with

$$q'(y, x_1, x_2, o_2, x_3) \equiv q'(y, x_1, o_2) \tag{11.6}$$

Then the missing value mechanism does *not* satisfy the MAR assumption, because for example

$$P(O_2 = 1, O_3 = 0|Y = y, X_1 = x_1, X_2 = x_2, X_3 = x_3) = q(y, x_1, x_3) \cdot (1 - q'(y, x_1, 1))$$

Nevertheless, estimation of the regression parameter is possible based on

$$f(y, x_1, z_2, z_3) \propto \begin{cases} q(y, x_1, z_3) \cdot f_\beta(y|x_1, z_2) \cdot g(z_2, z_3|x_1) & \text{if } z_2 \neq ?, z_3 \neq ? \\ q(y, x_1, z_3) \int f_\beta(y|x_1, x_2) g(x_2, z_3|x_1) \, dx_2 & \text{if } z_2 = ?, z_3 \neq ? \\ f_\beta(y|x_1, z_2) \cdot \int q(y, x_1, x_3) \cdot g(z_2, x_3|x_1) \, dx_3 & \text{if } z_2 \neq ?, z_3 = ? \\ \int\int q(y, x_1, x_3) \cdot f_\beta(y|x_1, x_2) \cdot g(x_2, x_3|x_1) \, dx_2 \, dx_3 & \text{if } z_2 = ?, z_3 = ? \end{cases}$$

The conditional distribution $g(x_2, x_3|x_1)$ and the observation probabilities $q(y, x_1, x_3)$ are to be parametrized and/or estimated nonparametrically. The estimation of $q(y, x_1, x_3)$ can be just based on the observed missing pattern for X_2; we have to solve the problem of a regression of O_2 on Y, X_1 and X_3. The additional missing values in X_3 cause no unsolvable problem, as the MAR assumption is satisfied because of (11.6).

12. Further Examples

The following examples should illustrate some methodological issues in the application of methods to handle missing values in the covariates. In the first example the application of ML estimation allows a substantial gain in the precision relative to a Complete Case Analysis, but doubts of the validity of the MAR assumption require a sensitivity analysis. In the second example a Complete Case Analysis gives a somewhat dubious result and we have to examine, whether this result is a methodological artifact.

12.1 Example 1: Risk factors for subsequent contralateral breast cancer

In a cohort of 56540 women with invasive breast cancer a nested case control study was conducted to investigate the role of radiation in the development of subsequent contralateral breast cancer (Storm et al. 1992). Cases were 529 women who developed contralateral breast cancer 8 or more years after first diagnosis. Controls were women with primary breast cancer who did not develop contralateral breast cancer. One control was matched to each case patient on the basis of age, calendar year of initial breast cancer diagnosis and survival time. Radiation dose to the contralateral breast was estimated for each patient on the basis of radiation measurement; for 16 cases and 13 controls radiotherapy status was unknown. Additionally, data were abstracted from the medical records on some potential risk factors for breast cancer. We focus our attention to the risk factors parity, family history of breast cancer and menopausal status. The distribution and the missing rates of these risk factors and of exposure to radiation therapy are shown in Table 12.1 and Table 12.2. The population considered are the 1029 women with known radio therapy status. Knowledge about possible cases of breast cancer in family history is not available for half of the women, whereas the missing rates are moderate for parity and menopausal status.

variable	abbreviation	missing rates		
		overall	cases	controls
menopausal status	MENO	8.6%	8.8%	8.3%
family history of breast cancer	FAMH	50.1%	46.8%	53.3%
parity	PARI	18.1%	18.5%	17.6 %
exposure to radiation therapy	EXPO	0%	–	–

Table 12.1: Missing rates for four potential risk factors.

Statistical inference can be based on the fitting of a logistic regression model with the categorical covariates age and latency (built by division into three groups) and the four binary variables of Table 12.1. It remains to chose an appropriate method to handle missing values.

We start with Complete Case Analysis. Due to the high missing rate there remain only 453 women for this analysis, i.e. 56% of the data is lost. The analysis is based on 213 cases and 240

variable	category	frequency absolute	frequency relative
MENO	1≙premenopausal	394	41.9%
	2≙postmenopausal	547	58.1%
FAMH	1≙without⎱ ⎰ breast cancer	425	82.8%
	2≙with ⎰ ⎱ in family history	88	17.2%
PARI	1≙no children	215	25.5%
	2≙one or more children	628	74.5%
EXPO	1≙unexposed	157	18.0%
	2≙exposed	872	82.0%

Table 12.2: Distribution of four potential risk factors.

controls, i.e., controls are slightly over-represented. The resulting estimates of the regression parameters for the four covariates of interest are shown in the upper part of Table 12.3.

Due to the high missing rate Complete Case Analysis seems not to be an appropriate method. We try next ML Estimation under the MAR assumption. As shown in Section 9.1, this requires to choose a parametric model to describe the distribution of the covariates. We use a log-linear model with interactions between all pairs of covariates. The resulting estimates are

		EXPO	PARI	FAMH	MENO
Complete	$\hat{\beta}$	-0.141	-0.581	0.591	-0.549
Case	$\widehat{sdv}(\hat{\beta})$	0.266	0.218	0.264	0.273
Analysis	95% CI	[-0.662,0.379]	[-1.008,-0.153]	[0.073,1.109]	[-1.084,-0.015]
ML	$\hat{\beta}$	0.037	-0.365	0.513	-0.263
estimation	$\widehat{sdv}(\hat{\beta})$	0.177	0.162	0.245	0.184
under MAR	95% CI	[-0.310,0.384]	[-0.681,-0.048]	[0.033,0.992]	[-0.624,0.098]

Table 12.3: Estimates and confidence intervals for the regression parameters based on a Complete Case Analysis and on ML estimation under the Missing At Random assumption.

shown in the lower part of Table 12.3. Compared to the results of the Complete Case Analysis the standards errors are now smaller for the effects of exposure, parity and menopausal status, as many subjects neglected in the Complete Case Analysis carry information on the relation of these variables to the occurrence of subsequent contralateral breast cancer. For the precision of the estimate of the effect of family history such an improvement could not be expected. The differences between the effect estimates of the Complete Case Analysis and the ML estimates are remarkable, we will discuss this point later.

ML estimation under the MAR assumption is also not a completely convincing approach here, as the MAR assumption is probably violated. Especially for the covariate family history of breast cancer we conjecture that the absence of cases of breast cancer in the family history results more often in a missing value than its presence. But also for menopausal status and parity the MAR assumption may be violated. Hence a sensitivity analysis as proposed in Chapter 8 is indicated here. However, the approaches of Chapter 8 cannot be directly applied, as they are restricted to missing values in one covariate. A generalization can be achieved using the following framework.

The basic task is to find a parametrization of the missing value mechanism, which allows us to specify alternatives to the MAR assumption. Let $X = (X_1, \ldots, X_p)$ be the vector of covariates. The missing value mechanism is described by the probabilities

$$q(M|y, x) := P(\{j|Z_j =?\} = M|Y = y, X = x) .$$

We start with the saturated log-linear model for the conditional missingness probabilities, i.e.,

$$q(M|y, x) = \prod_{S \subseteq M} \exp(\delta_S^{y,x}) .$$

We assume that the interaction parameters $\delta_S^{y,x}$ with $|S| \geq 2$ are independent of y and x, and that the main effects $\delta_{\{j\}}^{y,x}$ depend only on x_j and additionally on y and the completely observable covariates $X_A := (X_1, X_2, X_3)$, i.e. age, latency and exposure. We further decompose the main effects according to

$$\exp(\delta_{\{j\}}^{y,x}) = \exp(\gamma_{\{j\}}^{y,x_A}) \cdot MOR_{\{j\}}^{y,x_A}(x_j) . \tag{12.1}$$

Then

$$q(M|y, x) = \frac{\prod_{j \in M} \exp(\gamma_{\{j\}}^{y,x_A}) \cdot MOR_{\{j\}}^{y,x_A}(x_j) \cdot \prod_{S \subseteq M, |S| \geq 2} \exp(\gamma_S)}{\sum_{M' \subseteq \bar{A}} \left[\prod_{j \in M'} \exp(\gamma_{\{j\}}^{y,x_A}) \cdot MOR_{\{j\}}^{y,x_A}(x_i) \cdot \prod_{S \subseteq M', |S| \geq 2} \exp(\gamma_S) \right]}$$

such that

$$MOR_{\{j\}}^{y,x_A}(k) = \frac{P(Z_j =?|H(y, x_A,), X_j = k)}{P(Z_j \neq?|H(y, x_A), X_j = k)} \bigg/ \frac{P(Z_j =?|H(y, x_A), X = 1)}{P(Z_j \neq?|H(y, x_A), X_j = 1)}$$

where $H(y, x_A)$ denotes any event with $Y = y$, $X_A = x_A$, an arbitrary missing pattern of $(Z_{j'})_{j' \neq j}$ and arbitrary values of $(X_{j'})_{j' \neq j, j' \notin A}$. Hence $MOR_{\{j\}}^{y,x_A}(k)$ is the missingness odds ratio of the k-th category of X_j with respect to missingness of X_j, given $Y = y$, $X_A = x_A$, any arbitrary missing pattern and any true values of the remaining components. To keep the number of parameters $\gamma_{\{j\}}^{y,x_A}$ feasible we decompose $\gamma_{\{j\}}^{y,x_A}$ into

$$\gamma_{\{j\}}^{y,x_A} = \gamma_{\{j\}}^y + \sum_{i \in A} \gamma_{\{j\},i}^{x_i} + \sum_{i \in A} \gamma_{\{j\},i}^{y,x_i} \tag{12.2}$$

with restrictions $\gamma_{\{j\},i}^{x_i} = 0$ if $x_i = 1$ and $\gamma_{\{j\},i}^{y,x_i} = 0$ if $y = 0$ or $x_i = 1$. If all the missingness odds ratios are specified the regression parameter β can now be estimated jointly with the nuisance parameters by the ML principle. If all the missingness odds ratios are specified as 1.0, the missing value mechanism satisfies the MAR assumption.

The above framework allows to specify missingness odds ratios which are different between cases and controls, and which may depend on completely observable covariates. In the first steps we consider missingness odds ratios which are independent from y and x_A such that we have to specify one missingness odds ratio for each of the covariates parity, family history and menopausal status. We start with varying the logarithm of each single missingness odds ratio between -2 and 2 and observe the variation of the regression parameter estimates and their confidence intervals (Table 12.4). Only the variation of the missingness odds ratio of family history shows a substantial impact on the variation of the estimates, but mainly on the estimate of the effect of family history itself. We have mentioned above the strong conjecture that the presence of cases of breast cancer in family history is better known than its absence, i.e. we can assume that the missingness odds ratio for family history is less than 1. Under this restriction, we observe only larger estimates for the effect of family history than under the MAR assumption (5th line of Table 12.4). The same can be observed, if we consider the joint variation of the missingness odds ratios (6th line of Table 12.4).

So far we have assumed that the missingness odds ratios do not depend on the case-control status. To weaken this assumption we conducted two further sensitivity analyses, where the logarithms of the missingness odds ratio for family history show a ratio of $1 : 2$ between cases and controls, and vice versa, such that the logarithms vary between -2 and 0 for one group and between -1 and 0 for the other. The missingness odds ratios for the other two covariates vary between -2 and 2, and all combinations are considered. The results are shown in the fifth and sixth row of Table 6. The estimates for exposure, menopausal status and parity are again stable, but we have to recognize that the effect of family history diminishes, if the variation of the missingness probabilities is larger within cases than within controls. It seems to be hard to decide, whether this is probably true or wrong.

We arrive at the following conclusions, even if we allow some (plausible) violations of the MAR assumption: Parity has to be considered as a statistically significant risk factor at the 5% level (as its 95% confidence intervals never include 0); postmenopausal status is probably a preventive factor, but does not reach statistical significance; breast cancer in family history may increase the risk for secondary breast cancer, but the magnitude of this effect can be hardly determined from this data, because for doing this it is necessary to know the relation of the missingness odds ratios between cases and controls; there is no evidence for an effect of radiation with an odds ratio larger than 1.5, as the upper limit of the 95% confidence interval is always smaller.

We believe that the above analysis is adequate for this data set. It remains to discuss some methodological issues. The framework for a sensitivity analysis presented above is only one of several possible solutions. The basic problem is the modeling of a relation between several binary, correlated variables and some covariates. This problem is well known in statistics (cf. the overview of Zeger & Liang 1992). One may criticize the approach above, because the true value of a covariate affected with missing values is not allowed to influence the occurrence of

Variation of log(MOR)				Observed variation of the esimates of			
PARI	FAME	MENO		EXPO	PARI	FAMH	MENO
0	0	0	$\hat{\beta}$	0.037	-0.365	0.513	-0.263
0	0	0	95% CI	[-0.310,0.384]	[-0.681,-0.048]	[0.033,0.992]	[-0.624,0.098]
-2··2	0	0	$\hat{\beta}$	0.034 0.038	-0.367 -0.332	0.512 0.515	-0.266 -0.263
-2··2	0	0	95% CI	[-0.313,0.385]	[-0.683,-0.032]	[0.032,0.994]	[-0.628,0.099]
0	-2··2	0	$\hat{\beta}$	0.034 0.043	-0.387 -0.358	0.321 0.579	-0.264 -0.253
0	-2··2	0	95% CI	[-0.315,0.388]	[-0.703,-0.041]	[-0.085,1.042]	[-0.624,0.106]
0	0	-2··2	$\hat{\beta}$	0.035 0.038	-0.365 -0.364	0.511 0.515	-0.273 -0.243
0	0	-2··2	95% CI	[-0.312,0.384]	[-0.681,-0.048]	[0.032,0.995]	[-0.628,0.107]
0	-2··0	0	$\hat{\beta}$	0.037 0.043	-0.364 -0.358	0.513 0.579	-0.264 -0.263
0	-2··0	0	95% CI	[-0.310,0.388]	[-0.681,-0.042]	[0.033,1.042]	[-0.624,0.098]
-2··2	-2··0	-2··2	$\hat{\beta}$	0.033 0.046	-0.369 -0.336	0.510 0.592	-0.280 -0.236
-2··2	-2··0	-2··2	95% CI	[-0.314,0.391]	[-0.684,-0.011]	[0.031,1.055]	[-0.632,0.112]
-2··2	-1··0 for cases	-2··2	$\hat{\beta}$	0.032 0.041	-0.369 -0.317	0.511 0.802	-0.282 -0.239
-2··2	-2··0 for controls	-2··2	95% CI	[-0.316,0.387]	[-0.684,-0.005]	[0.031,1.268]	[-0.637,0.112]
-2··2	-1··0 for cases	-2··2	$\hat{\beta}$	0.032 0.048	-0.369 -0.322	0.341 0.556	-0.276 -0.234
-2··2	-2··0 for controls	-2··2	95% CI	[-0.314,0.392]	[-0.684,-0.021]	[-0.128,0.994]	[-0.631,0.113]

Table 12.4: For each analysis the smallest and largest estimate for $\hat{\beta}$ and the smallest lower bound and the largest upper bound of the confidence intervals are given.

missing values in another. To avoid this, we can use instead of (12.1) and (12.2)

$$\exp(\delta_{\{j\}}^{y,x}) = \exp(\gamma_{\{j\}}^{y,x\overline{\{j\}}}) \cdot MOR_{\{j\}}^{y,x\overline{\{j\}}}(x_j)$$

and

$$\gamma_{\{j\}}^{y,x'} = \gamma_{\{j\}}^{y} + \sum_{i \neq j} \gamma_{\{j\},i}^{x'} + \sum_{i \neq j} \gamma_{\{j\},i}^{y,x'}$$

with a few more parameters. However, specifying all *MOR*s as 1, we now do not arrive at the MAR assumption. A rigid alternative to the use of log-linear model to describe the joint distribution of the missing indicators would be the use of marginal models. We should also mention that maximization of the likelihood causes some numerical problems, due to the large number of parameters (70 parameters in this example). Our computations are based on the Newton-Raphson method and it is essential to use appropriate start values to avoid numerical singularity of the matrix of second derivatives. We derive start values from the complete case estimates of the regression parameters and of the parameters of the log-linear model for the covariates and from the estimates of γ under the MAR assumption. Numerical problems to estimate the nuisance parameters also prevent to consider all 1058 women. Further aspects of this approach to investigate violations of the MAR assumption are considered in Vach & Blettner (1994).

Although we do not want to recommend the use of (Unconditional) Probability Imputation and Additional Category, we have applied them to this data set. The results are shown in Table 12.5. There are no large differences between the estimates of Probability Imputation or Additional Category compared to ML estimation, which can be partially explained by the fact that all pairwise correlations between the covariates are small. The negative estimate for the additional category of family history requires an explanation, as the effect of family history is positive. This explanation is given by the difference of the missing rates between cases and controls shown in Table 12.1, which implies that in the subgroup represented by the additional category controls are more frequent than cases. Finally it should be mentioned that the estimates for the standard errors of the effect of menopausal status seem to be too small for Probability Imputation and Additional Category.

It remains to give some remarks on the discrepancy between the estimates of the Complete Case Analysis and the estimates of ML Estimation. We have shown in Section 4.4 and 9.4 that the results of a Complete Case analysis can be substantially biased. However, the basic supposition for this is a dependence of the missing rates on the outcome variable in combination with a dependence on some covariates. An analysis of the missing rates and the parameters $\gamma_{\{j\}}^{y,x_i}$ give no hints that this supposition is valid here. As we can exclude this source of bias, the observed discrepancies may give a hint that restriction to subjects without missing values means a selection of a subgroup, where the effects of menopausal status and parity are really larger. As this would be of great interest for the epidemiologists, it is worth to investigate, whether such a hint can be really seen in these discrepancies. We have to answer the basic question, whether a random reduction of the complete population to 213 cases and 240 controls can explain the discrepancies. To give a first answer, we reduce the population after imputation of unconditional relative frequencies 100 times and count, how often the resulting estimates for parity and menopausal status are smaller than -0.581 or -0.549, respectively. These frequencies are 14 and 5. Hence it seems not to be justified to look for a deep interpretation of these discrepancies.

		EXPO	PARI	FAMH	MENO
Complete Case	$\hat{\beta}$	-0.141	-0.581	0.591	-0.549
Analysis	$\widehat{sdv}(\hat{\beta})$	0.266	0.218	0.264	0.273
ML Estimation	$\hat{\beta}$	0.037	-0.365	0.513	-0.263
under MAR	$\widehat{sdv}(\hat{\beta})$	0.177	0.162	0.245	0.184
Probability	$\hat{\beta}$	0.047	-0.379	0.528	-0.301
Imputation	$\widehat{sdv}(\hat{\beta})$	0.177	0.161	0.241	0.177
Additional	$\hat{\beta}$	0.049	-0.337	0.508	-0.293
Category	$\widehat{sdv}(\hat{\beta})$	0.176	0.161	0.243	0.177
	$\hat{\beta}_{AC}$		-0.100	-0.204	-0.126
	$\widehat{sdv}(\hat{\beta}_{AC})$		0.216	0.136	0.260

Table 12.5: Comparison of the results of Complete Case Analysis, ML Estimation under MAR, Probability Imputation and Additional Category.

12.2 Example 2: A study on the role of DNA content for the prognosis of ovarian cancer patients

In a group of 205 patients treated for ovarian cancer the role of DNA content as a prognostic factor was examined (Pfisterer et al., unpublished). Besides ploidy status (categorized as diploid and aneuploid tumors using a cut point of 1.1) and S-phase fraction the prognostic factors age, FIGO stage, grade of malignancy and residual tumor after primary surgery were considered. Data are nearly complete for all factors except S-phase fraction. The missing rate of S-phase fraction is low (8%) for patients with diploid tumors but very high (73%) for patients with aneuploid tumors (Table 12.6). This reflects a well known problem in the exact assessment of S-phase fractions in aneuploid tissue. Additionally, the distribution of S-phase differs substantially in the two ploidy groups. We analyse the prognostic value of the S phase fraction by comparing Kaplan-Meier-estimates between the groups defined by S-phase fraction <7%, 7%-12% and >12%. As shown in Figure 12.1, for diploid patients no effect of S-phase fraction can be observed, whereas aneuploid patients show smaller survival times with increasing S-fraction. We further conduct a Complete Case Analysis for a proportional hazard model with the additional covariates age, stage and residual tumors. It shows a significant interaction between ploidy status and S-phase fraction (p=0.039).

One may argue that this discrepancy between subjects with diploid and aneuploid tumors is an artifact due to the variation of the missing rates. Additionally one may conjecture that observability of S-phase fraction is related to its true value, i.e., that the MAR assumption is violated. However, both conjectures are irrelevant, as a Complete Case Analysis is robust against any dependence of observation probabilities on the covariates (see Section 9.4). A dependence of the observability on the outcome variable is theoretically possible here, as the DNA content was measured retrospectively from paraffin-embedded tissues, but it is not

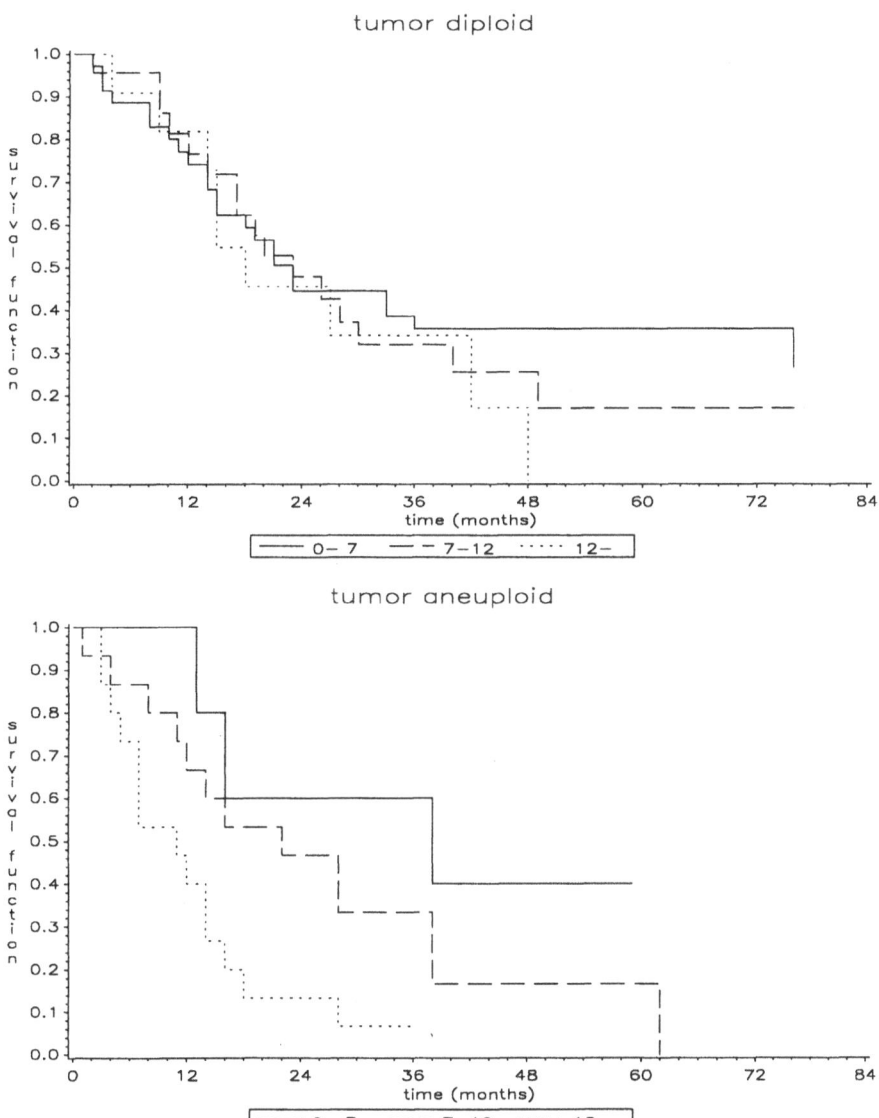

Figure 12.1: Kaplan Meier estimates of survival time for patients with low, medium and high S-phase fractions. Upper Part: Patients with diploid tumors. Lower Part: Patients with Aneuploid tumors.

	S-phase fraction				
	<7%	7%-12%	>12%	?	Total
diploid	35	24	11	6	76
aneuploid	5	15	15	94	129

	S-phase fraction		
	<7%	7%-12%	>12%
diploid	50%	34%	16%
aneuploid	14%	43%	43%

Table 12.6: Distribution of S-phase fraction. Upper Part: Absolute Frequencies. Lower Part: Relative Frequency within subjects with observed S-phase fraction.

probable. It is also rather difficult to find a plausible explanation based on the existence of unknown prognostic factors related to the dependence of the observability of S-phase fraction on the ploidy status. Hence we have little reason to distrust the results of the Complete Case Analysis. For the examination of the prognostic value of S-phase fraction we cannot expect any improvement from more sophisticated methods to handle missing values, as the covariate S-phase fraction is the covariate affected with missing values. The subjects neglected in the complete case analysis carry no information of interest.

13. Discussion

Missing values in the covariates are a challenge in the daily work of statisticians. The standard approach of most statistical software packages is the Complete Case Analysis. Most statisticians follow this suggestion although they feel that there must be more efficient ways. Hence many readers of this book will look for a list recommending better methods. Based on the investigations of this book such an attempt will be made in the next two sections. However, there exists not (yet) a general standard technique to handle missing values in the covariates, but we are able to distinguish some (new) methods with good and some (old) methods with bad statistical properties. The presented difficulties to give general recommendations also highlight some important issues of future research. Additional topics are summarized in the third section, and the book finishes with an important remark.

Whenever we are confronted with missing values we have first to ask whether we can exclude a relation between the true, unobserved values and their observability. If we can exclude this, the *Missing At Random* (MAR) assumption is satisfied, and it makes sense to think about sophisticated methods to handle missing values which are superior to Complete Case Analysis. This is the topic of the first section. If the MAR assumption is violated, our first aim should be to avoid a biased estimation due to this violation. This is the topic of the second section.

13.1 Statistical Inference if the MAR Assumption is Satisfied

The first important remark: The regression parameter estimates of a Complete Case Analysis are not always consistent for the true parameters. They can be asymptotically biased if the probability for the occurrence of a missing value is related to the outcome variable. This can be usually excluded for studies with a prospective scheme of data collection, but it is typical for studies with a retrospective scheme, especially for case control studies. In this situation it is possible to asses the bias by a simple computation based on the observed missing rates (see Section 4.4). If this indicates a biased estimation you should use one of the sophisticated methods mentioned later.

Otherwise, before thinking about methods to overcome a potential inefficiency of Complete Case Analysis one should investigate whether in your particular application a gain in efficiency can be really expected. For example if we have two covariates where only the second is affected by missing values, we cannot expect any improvement in estimating the effect of the second covariate. We can expect a gain in precision to estimate the effect of the first covariate, but this may not imply the use of sophisticated methods. It may be sufficient to omit the second covariate, because then in estimating the effect of the first covariate we can use the complete sample to increase precision. However, in general this estimate is biased, but this bias may be negligible if the covariates are not correlated or if the correlation is small. Hence in many situations the use of sophisticated methods may be only necessary if we are interested in the effect of a covariate with no or a few missing values and if the effect of this covariate is subject to be confounded by the effect of a covariate with substantially more missing values.

Methods to fill the gaps in your data by imputation of means or by regarding missing values as an additional category cannot be recommended. They are often associated with a serious bias and a substantial underestimation of the variance (see Sections 4.5, 4.6, 5.8 and 7.1). Imputation based on estimates conditioned on the observed covariates seems to be the best among these bad methods, but also this approach cannot be recommended in general (see Sections 4.6, 5.9 and 6.3). For logistic regression with categorical covariates there exists a simple method called Filling to achieve consistent estimates of the regression parameters, but standard errors are not directly available (see Section 4.3).

If you are really looking for good methods to handle missing values, maximum likelihood estimation should be your first choice. Then you are sure to get efficient estimates. The disadvantage is the necessity to specify the joint distribution of the covariates at least in part. If all covariates are categorical loglinear models provide a tool which seems to be flexible enough for this task (see Sections 10.1 and 12.1). For continuous covariates parametric assumptions like a joint multivariate normal distribution are usually too restrictive. In addition computation of the ML estimates causes more difficulties. There are approaches to overcome the necessity to specify a parametric family by using nonparametric estimates. In this book Semiparametric ML Estimation (Sections 4.2 and 9.2) and Estimation of the Score Function (Sections 4.3 and 9.3) have been considered. However, so far they have been only considered for the case of two covariates where one is affected by missing values, and generalizations for constellations of practical interest are cumbersome. None of the sophisticated methods is implemented in standard statistical software packages.

13.2 Statistical Inference if the MAR Assumption is Questionable

If the MAR assumption is in doubt, Complete Case Analysis should be the first choice, because violation of the MAR assumption does not destroy consistency of the regression parameters. Exceptions occur in settings where the estimates would be not consistent even if the MAR assumption is valid, cf. the last section. It seems to be very difficult to get estimates superior to those of a Complete Case Analysis except if one has a rather precise knowledge of the type of violation. In this situation one can estimate the regression parameters under a prespecified missing value mechanism not satisfying the MAR assumption. Additionally we can try several non-MAR mechanisms such that we conduct an analysis to which degree an estimate may be sensitive against violations of the MAR assumption (see Chapter 8 and Section 12.1).

It is often supposed that there exists something like a critical missing rate up to which missing values are not too dangerous. The believe in such a global missing rate is rather stupid. Moreover, all investigations in this book demonstrate that the variation of the missing rates among subgroups is the key to relevant statistical properties of any method to handle missing values. This concerns the bias of Complete Case Analysis and other ad hoc methods as well as the efficiency of sophisticated methods.

Independent of the methods used missing values and a possible violation of the MAR assumption may have some impact on the results of statistical inference. Hence in any publication missing rates should be reported in detail and the possible implications on the results should be discussed.

13.3 Topics of Future Research

Further Development of Methods

The main gap to be filled is the lack of a general method to handle missing continuous covariates with arbitrary missing patterns. It seems to be cumbersome to generalize Semi-parametric ML estimation and the Estimation of the Score Function without restricting the full nonparametric handling of the distribution of the covariates. Parametric approaches more flexible than the multivariate normal distribution may be acceptable, even if there is a danger of misspecification, because our aim is to estimate mixing distributions and it seems to be sufficient to approximate roughly the mean and variance structure of these distributions. Similar it may be sufficient to get a crude estimate for the correction of variance due to estimation of the mixing distributions as the portion of this correction at the total variance is in most cases small (cf. Section 5.10).

Most methods developed so far are restricted to regression models specified by a full likelihood. There is a demand to generalize them for models based on weaker specifications, especially generalized linear models, the Cox proportional hazards model, conditional logistic regression, models for longitudinal data and generalized additive models.

Finally the development should result in computer programs available for the statistical community. It may be controversial to add programs for methods requiring the MAR assumption to popular statistical software packages. We have to expect that these programs will be used more often in situations where the MAR assumption is violated than in situations where it is valid, cf. Vach (1994).

Efficiency and Semiparametric Estimation

Although we may be glad if we have some general method to handle missing values in a manner superior to Complete Case Analysis there remains a demand for optimal methods. The efficiency comparisons between ML Estimation, Pseudo ML Estimation and Filling in Chapter 5 have highlighted some issues: The choice of the non-parametric procedure as a part of a semiparametric approach may be crucial; semiparametric approaches may be as efficient as a parametric approach for some missing value mechanisms, for others the same approach may show a substantial loss; semiparametric approaches need not to be more efficient than Complete Case Analysis. On the other side the general theory of semiparametric estimation provides us with a lot of results on optimality (e.g. Pfanzagl 1990, Newey 1990). First steps to connect these results with missing data problems are given by Schick & Susarla (1988) and Robins & Rotnitzky (1992).

Violation of the MAR assumption

Although the MAR assumption is highly questionable in many applications little is known about the sensitivity of estimators against violations of the MAR assumption. In this book we presented a suggestion to investigate the sensitivity of a single estimate (Chapter 8) and application of this procedure to examples suggest that in general estimators are rather robust against violations of the MAR assumption if the degree of violation do not depend on the outcome variable or on other covariates (cf. also Section 12.1). A similar conjecture is expressed by Schemper & Smith (1990). Computations of the asymptotic bias by Illi (1993) substantiate this conjecture. This question requires further investigation and conditions restricting the possible bias to a negligible magnitude are desirable.

Multiple Imputation Methods

The approaches considered in this book are more or less in the tradition of parametric statistics. A further class of approaches is characterized by processing multiple imputations for the missing values and summarizing the resulting estimates. This approach is widespread in the analysis of survey data (Rubin 1987). A first result for a unifying view to these two classes of methods is given by Reilly & Pepe (1993a,1993b): The estimates of a Hot-Deck multiple imputation procedure with infinite number of repetitions are asymptotically equivalent to those of the Mean Score Method. However, multiple imputation methods and semiparametric approaches share the problem to handle conditional distributions which is cumbersome for more than two covariates with arbitrary missing patterns (see Chapter 10).

Missing Values and the Design of Studies

In planing a data collection procedure we often know in advance which variables will be affected by missing values and which not. So the situation is similar to measurement error problems where we know in advance which variables can only be regarded as a surrogate measure. Validation sampling and repeated measurements are two approaches to achieve valid statistical inference in spite of measurement error (cf. for example Willett (1989) and Marshall (1989)). Similar approaches can be also used to improve the handling of missing values, especially if the MAR assumption is questionable. Subsampling of the nonresponders is one approach (see Section 11.3). Another idea is the sampling of surrogate variables which may be less affected by missing values. These issues should be paid more attention in future.

13.4 Final Remark

Even the nicest results about methods to handle missing values should not seduce us to forget that they are never a substitute for complete data. The MAR assumption is doubtful in many applications, and hence missing values are often a source of misleading results. If the MAR assumption can be maintained, there remains a loss of efficiency. The effort in propagating the progress in the development of statistical methods to handle missing values should always be smaller than the effort in propagating the importance of completely measured data.

Appendix A.1

ML Estimation in the presence of missing values

Let be $V = (V_1, \ldots, V_k)$ a k-variate random variable with density $f_\xi^V(v)$. The observability of the single components is described by indicator variables O_i and $O := (O_1, \ldots, O_k)$. The conditional distribution of O given V, i.e., the missing value mechanism, is given by the conditional probabilities $p_q(o|u) := P(O = o|V = v)$. q is the parameter describing the missing value mechanism. The random variable we really observe is $Z = (Z_1, \ldots, Z_k)$ with

$$Z_i = \begin{cases} V_i & \text{if } O_i = 1 \\ ? & \text{otherwise} \end{cases}.$$

Maximum likelihood estimation requires the density of Z, evaluated at the observed value of Z. This density is achieved by evaluating the marginal density of the joint distribution of O and the observed components of V at the observed values, i.e., we have to integrate the density of the joint distribution of O and V over the unobserved components of V.

Although it is easy to express this by words, it is somewhat technical to describe it by a formula. For a possible outcome z of Z we define

$$M(z) := \{i \in \{1, \ldots, k\} \mid z_i = ?\} \text{ and } \bar{M}(z) := \{i \in \{1, \ldots, k\} \mid z_i \neq ?\}$$

indicating the missing and the non-missing components. Further we regard O as a function $o(z)$ of Z, and similar the observed components of V as a function $v(Z)$ with

$$v(z)(i) = z_i \text{ for } i \in \bar{M}(z),$$

whereas the remaining components are not defined. Then

$$f_{\xi,q}^Z(z) = \int p_q(o(z)|v(z)) f_\xi^V(v(z)) dv_{M(z)}.$$

This result is often expressed (e.g. Little & Rubin 1987, p.89) as

$$f_{\xi,q}^{V_{\bar{M}}}(v_{\bar{M}(z)}) = \int p_q(o|v_M, v_{\bar{M}}) f_\xi^V(v_M, v_{\bar{M}}) dv_M,$$

but note that it is somewhat difficult to regard $f_{\xi,q}^{V_{\bar{M}}}$ really as a density, because $V_{\bar{M}}$ is a random variable with a random number of components. The essential fact is that the contribution to the likelihood can be expressed as a marginal density evaluated at observed values.

In general, the distribution of Z depends jointly on ξ and q. The assumption

$$p_q(o|v) \equiv p_q(o|v_{\bar{M}}) \quad \text{for all } M \subseteq \{1, \ldots, k\} \text{ and for all } o \text{ with } o(i) = 0 \Leftrightarrow i \in M$$
(14.1)

obviously allows to decompose the density of Z, such that ML estimation can be based on

$$\int f_\xi^V(v(z)) dv_{M(z)},$$

i.e., we can now estimate ξ without further knowledge of the missing value mechanism. Because of this fact Rubin (1976) calls the assumption (14.1) *Missing at Random* (MAR).

Appendix A.2

The EM algorithm

General

The Expectation Maximization (EM) algorithm is a general tool to maximize a loglikelihood resulting from a marginal density, i.e., we have a density $f_\lambda(u,w)$ and the marginal density $f_\lambda(u) = \int f_\lambda(u,w)dw$, and we want to maximize $\ell(\lambda;u) := \log f_\lambda(u)$ over λ.

The idea of the EM algorithm is to start with an arbitrary guess λ^0 for λ, then to consider the conditional distribution of W given $U = u$, to compute in the E-step the expected loglikelihood $\int[\log f_\lambda(u,w)]f_{\lambda^0}(w|u)dw$, and to receive a new guess λ^1 by maximizing the expected loglikelihood over λ. Then these steps are iterated until convergence is reached.

It can be easily seen that this procedure increases $\ell(\lambda,u)$ in each step: Denoting

$$Q(\lambda,\lambda') := \int[\log f_\lambda(u,w)]f_{\lambda'}(w|u)dw$$

such that $\lambda \mapsto Q(\lambda,\lambda^t)$ is maximized in the t-th step, we have with $\ell(\lambda,u) = \log f_\lambda(u,w) - \log f_\lambda(w|u)$ and $H(\lambda,\lambda') := \int[\log f_\lambda(w|u)]f_{\lambda'}(w|u)dw$ the relation

$$\ell(\lambda^{t+1},u) - \ell(\lambda^t,u) = [Q(\lambda^{t+1},\lambda^t) - Q(\lambda^t,\lambda^t)] - [H(\lambda^{t+1},\lambda^t) - H(\lambda^t,\lambda^t)].$$

It can be shown that $\lambda \mapsto H(\lambda,\lambda')$ is maximized for $\lambda = \lambda'$, hence $Q(\lambda^{t+1},\lambda^t) \geq Q(\lambda^t,\lambda^t)$ implies $\ell(\lambda^{t+1},u) \geq \ell(\lambda^t,u)$. It is much more difficult to find conditions, which ensure the convergence of the EM algorithm to a local maximum. Some results can be find in Dempster, Laird & Rubin (1977) and Wu (1983).

Note that $f_\lambda(u)$ and $f_\lambda(u,w)$ need not to be densities. It is sufficient that $f_\lambda(u)f_\lambda(w|u) = f_\lambda(u,w)$ holds. Especially if $f_\lambda(u)$ and $f_\lambda(u,w)$ are only factors of a density, the EM algorithm works. In this setting it is used in our applications.

If we want to maximize a likelihood resulting from independent repetitions, the EM algorithm works on each single contribution, i.e., we maximize in the t-th step

$$\sum_{r=1}^{n} \int [\log f_\lambda(u_r,w)]f_{\lambda^t}(w|u_r)dw$$

Application in Missing Value Problems

ML estimation based on data with missing values is one of the main applications of the EM algorithm. In Appendix A.1 we have shown that the contribution of a unit with missing values in some components can be expressed as

$$\int f_\lambda(o,v_M,v_{\bar{M}})dv_M$$

with $\lambda = (\xi,q)$ and $f_\lambda(o,v_M,v_{\bar{M}}) = p_q(o|v_M,v_{\bar{M}})f_\xi^V(v_M,v_{\bar{M}})$. To apply the EM algorithm, we set $u := (o,v_{\bar{M}})$ and $w := v_M$, such that $f_\lambda(u,w) = f_\lambda(o,v) = p_q(o|v)f_\xi^V(v)$. Then in the

E-step the expected likelihood based on λ^t is

$$\int [\log p_q(o|v_M, v_{\bar{M}})] f_{\lambda^t}(v_M|o, v_{\bar{M}}) dv_M + \int [\log f_\xi^V(v_M, v_{\bar{M}})] f_{\lambda^t}(v_M|o, v_{\bar{M}}) dv_M \ .$$

If the MAR assumption holds, then ML estimation of ξ does not involve estimation of q, the contribution to the likelihood can be expressed as

$$\int f_\xi^V(v_M, v_{\bar{M}}) dv_M \ ,$$

and in the E-step of the EM algorithm the expected loglikelihood based on ξ^t is

$$\int [\log f_\xi^V(v_M, v_{\bar{M}})] f_\xi^V(v_M|v_{\bar{M}}) dv_M \ .$$

EM Algorithm and Variance Estimation

As we compute ordinary ML estimates, traditional theory allows estimation of the asymptotic variance via the Fisher information. Whereas the EM algorithm relates maximization of the incomplete data likelihood to maximization of the complete data likelihood, a basic result of Louis (1982) relates the Fisher information of the incomplete data likelihood to the complete data likelihood. He shows that

$$-\frac{\partial^2}{\partial\lambda\partial\lambda} \log f_\lambda(u)\Big|_{\lambda^0}$$

$$= \int \left(-\frac{\partial^2}{\partial\lambda\partial\lambda} \log f_\lambda(u,w)\Big|_{\lambda^0}\right) f_{\lambda^0}(w|u) dw - Var\left[\frac{\partial}{\partial\lambda} \log f_\lambda(u,W)\Big|_{\lambda^0}\Big| U = u\right]$$

which implies

$$E_{\lambda^0}\left(-\frac{\partial^2}{\partial\lambda\partial\lambda} \log f_\lambda(U)\Big|_{\lambda^0}\right)$$

$$= \int\int (-\frac{\partial^2}{\partial\lambda\partial\lambda} \log f_\lambda(u,w)\Big|_{\lambda^0} f_{\lambda^0}(w|u) f_{\lambda^0}(u) dw du$$

$$- \int Var\left[\frac{\partial}{\partial\lambda} \log f_\lambda(u,W)\Big|_{\lambda^0}\Big| U = u\right] f_{\lambda^0}(u) du$$

$$= E_{\lambda^0}\left(-\frac{\partial^2}{\partial\lambda\partial\lambda} \log f_\lambda(U,W)\Big|_{\lambda^0}\right) - E_{\lambda^0} H_{\lambda^0}(U)$$

with $H_{\lambda^0}(u) = Var\left[\frac{\partial}{\partial\lambda} \log f_\lambda(u,W)\Big|_{\lambda^0}\Big| U = u\right]$

i.e., the Fisher information of the incomplete data likelihood can be achieved by subtracting $E_{\lambda^0} H_{\lambda^0}(U)$ from the Fisher information of the complete data likelihood. If the M-Step of the EM algorithm allows the use of standard statistical software we often get also an estimate for the Fisher information of the complete data likelihood, and hence it remains only to subtract $E_{\lambda^0} H_{\lambda^0}(U)$.

Appendix B.1

Explicit Representation of the Score Function of ML Estimation and the Information Matrix in the Complete Data Case

The contribution of a single unit to the loglikelihood is

$$\ell^*(\beta; y, j, k) = \log[\mu_{jk}(\beta)^y (1 - \mu_{jk}(\beta))^{1-y}] \,.$$

In this sequel we omit the argument of μ_{jk}. The components of the score function $S_n^*(\beta)$ are

$$\frac{1}{n} \frac{\partial}{\partial \beta_s} \ell_n^*(\beta) = \frac{1}{n} \sum_{j=1}^{J} \sum_{k=1}^{K} n_{1jk} \frac{\mu_{jk}^s}{\mu_{jk}} - n_{0jk} \frac{\mu_{jk}^s}{1 - \mu_{jk}}$$

$$= \frac{1}{n} \sum_{j=1}^{J} \sum_{k=1}^{K} [n_{1jk}(1 - \Lambda_{jk}) - n_{0jk}\Lambda_{jk}] I(s \in \{0, 1j, 2k\})$$

with $\mu_{jk}^s := \dfrac{\partial}{\partial \beta_s} \mu_{jk} = \Lambda_{jk}(1 - \Lambda_{jk}) I(s \in \{0, 1j, 2k\})$ and $\Lambda_{jk} := \Lambda(\beta_0 + \beta_{1j} + \beta_{2k})$

and the components of the Fisher information matrix $I_{\beta\beta}^*(\beta, \pi, \tau)$ are

$$I_{\beta_s \beta_t}^*(\beta, \pi, \tau)$$

$$= \sum_{j=1}^{J} \sum_{k=1}^{K} -E\left[\frac{\partial^2}{\partial \beta_s \partial \beta_t} \ell^*(\beta; Y, j, k) \,\Big|\, X_1 = j, X_2 = k \right] \pi_{k|j} \tau_j$$

$$= \sum_{j=1}^{J} \sum_{k=1}^{K} \frac{\mu_{jk}^s \mu_{jk}^t}{\mu_{jk}(1 - \mu_{jk})} \pi_{k|j} \tau_j = \sum_{j=1}^{J} \sum_{k=1}^{K} \Lambda_{jk}(1 - \Lambda_{jk}) I(s, t \in \{0, 1j, 2k\}) \pi_{k|j} \tau_j \,.$$

Considering the joint estimation of $\theta = (\beta, \pi)$ in the complete data case, the contribution to the loglikelihood of a single unit is

$$\ell^*(\theta; y, j, k) = \ell^*(\beta; y, j, k) + \log \pi_{k|j}$$

and the partial derivative with respect to π is

$$\frac{\partial}{\partial \pi_{k'|j'}} \ell^*(\theta; y, j, k) = \begin{cases} 0 & \text{if } j \neq j' \\ -\frac{1}{\pi_{k|j}} & \text{if } j = j', k = k' \\ -\frac{1}{\pi_{1|j}} & \text{if } j = j', k = 1 \end{cases} \,.$$

The Fisher information matrix $I_{\theta\theta}^*(\xi)$ is a block diagonal matrix with blocks $I_{\beta\beta}^*(\xi)$ and $I_{\pi\pi}^*(\xi)$. The components of the latter are

$$I_{\pi_{k'|j'} \pi_{k''|j''}}^*(\beta, \pi, \tau) = \begin{cases} 0 & \text{if } j' \neq j'' \\ \left(\frac{1}{\pi_{1j}} + \frac{1}{\pi_{k|j}} \right) \tau_j & \text{if } j := j' = j'', k := k' = k'' \\ \frac{1}{\pi_{1|j}} \tau_j & \text{if } j := j' = j'', k' \neq k'' \end{cases} \,.$$

Appendix B.2

Explicit Representation of the Score Function of ML Estimation and the Information Matrix

The contribution of a single unit to the loglikelihood is

$$\ell^{ML}(\beta, \pi; y, j, k) = \begin{cases} \log[\mu_{jk}(\beta)^y(1 - \mu_{jk}(\beta))^{1-y}] + \log \pi_{k|j} & \text{if } k \neq ? \\ \log[\mu_{j?}(\beta, \pi)^y(1 - \mu_{j?}(\beta, \pi))^{1-y}] & \text{if } k = ? \end{cases}.$$

In this sequel we omit the arguments of μ_{jk} and $\mu_{j?}$. With $\Lambda'_{jk} := \Lambda_{jk}(1 - \Lambda_{jk})$ the partial derivates are

$$\frac{\partial}{\partial \beta_s} \ell^{ML}(\beta, \pi; 1, j, k) = \frac{\mu^s_{jk}}{\mu_{jk}}; \quad \frac{\partial}{\partial \beta_s} \ell^{ML}(\beta, \pi; 0, j, k) = -\frac{\mu^s_{jk}}{1 - \mu_{jk}}$$

$$\text{with } \mu^s_{jk} := \frac{\partial}{\partial \beta_s} \mu_{jk} = \begin{cases} \Lambda'_{jk} I(s \in \{0, 1j, 2k\}) & \text{if } k \neq ? \\ \sum_{k'=1}^K \pi_{k'|j} \Lambda'_{jk'} I(s \in \{0, 1j, 2k'\}) & \text{if } k = ? \end{cases}$$

and

$$\frac{\partial}{\partial \pi_{k'|j'}} \ell^{ML}(\beta, \pi; i, j, k) = \begin{cases} \frac{1}{\pi_{k|j}} & \text{if } j = j', k \neq ?, k = k' \\ -\frac{1}{\pi_{1|j}} & \text{if } j = j', k \neq ?, k = 1 \\ \frac{\mu_{jk'} - \mu_{j1}}{\mu_{j?}} & \text{if } j = j', k = ?, i = 1 \\ -\frac{\mu_{jk'} - \mu_{j1}}{1 - \mu_{j?}} & \text{if } j = j', k = ?, i = 0 \\ 0 & \text{otherwise} \end{cases},$$

and the second partial derivates are

$$\frac{\partial^2}{\partial \beta_s \partial \beta_t} \ell^{ML}(\beta, \pi; 1, j, k) = \frac{\mu^{st}_{jk} \mu_{jk} - \mu^s_{jk} \mu^t_{jk}}{\mu^2_{jk}}$$

$$\frac{\partial^2}{\partial \beta_s \partial \beta_t} \ell^{ML}(\beta, \pi; 0, j, k) = -\frac{\mu^{st}_{jk}(1 - \mu_{jk}) + \mu^s_{jk} \mu^t_{jk}}{(1 - \mu_{jk})^2}$$

$$\frac{\partial^2}{\partial \beta_s \partial \pi_{k'|j'}} \ell^{ML}(\beta, \pi; i, j, k) = \begin{cases} \frac{(\mu^s_{jk'} - \mu^s_{j1})\mu_{j?} - (\mu_{jk'} - \mu_{j1})\mu^s_{j?}}{(\mu_{j?})^2} & \text{if } j = j', k = ?, i = 1 \\ -\frac{(\mu^s_{jk'} - \mu^s_{j1})(1 - \mu_{j?}) + (\mu_{jk'} - \mu_{j1})\mu^s_{j?}}{(1 - \mu_{j?})^2} & \text{if } j = j', k = ?, i = 0 \\ 0 & \text{otherwise} \end{cases}$$

$$\frac{\partial^2}{\partial \pi_{k'|j'} \partial \pi_{k''|j''}} \ell^{ML}(\beta, \pi; i, j, k) = \begin{cases} -\frac{1}{\pi^2_{k|j}} & \text{if } j = j' = j'', k \neq ?, k = k' = k'' \\ -\frac{1}{\pi^2_{1|j}} & \text{if } j = j' = j'', k \neq ?, k = 1 \\ -\frac{(\mu_{jk'} - \mu_{j1})(\mu_{jk''} - \mu_{j1})}{(\mu_{j?})^2} & \text{if } j = j' = j'', k = ?, i = 1 \\ -\frac{(\mu_{jk'} - \mu_{j1})(\mu_{jk''} - \mu_{j1})}{(1 - \mu_{j?})^2} & \text{if } j = j' = j'', k = ?, i = 0 \\ 0 & \text{otherwise} \end{cases}$$

with $\mu_{jk}^{st} := \dfrac{\partial^2}{\partial \beta_s \partial \beta_t} \mu_{jk}$

$$= \begin{cases} \Lambda_{jk}'' I(s \in \{0, 1j, 2k\}) I(t \in \{0, 1j, 2k\}) & \text{if } k \neq ? \\ \sum_{k'=1}^{K} \pi_{k'|j} \Lambda_{jk'}'' I(s \in \{0, 1j, 2k'\}) \} I(t \in \{0, 1j, 2k'\}) & \text{if } k = ? \end{cases}.$$

and $\Lambda_{jk}'' := \Lambda_{jk}(1 - \Lambda_{jk})(1 - 2\Lambda_{jk})$

The components of the score function $S_{ML}^n(\beta, \pi)$ are now

$$\frac{1}{n} \frac{\partial}{\partial \beta_s} \ell_{ML}^n(\beta, \pi) = \frac{1}{n} \sum_{j=1}^{J} \sum_{k=1}^{K+1} (n_{1jk} \frac{\mu_{jk}^s}{\mu_{jk}} - n_{0jk} \frac{\mu_{jk}^s}{1 - \mu_{jk}})$$

$$= \frac{1}{n} \sum_{j=1}^{J} \left[\sum_{k=1}^{K} [n_{1jk}(1 - \Lambda_{jk}) - n_{0jk} \Lambda_{jk}] I(s \in \{0, 1j, 2k\}) \right.$$

$$\left. + n_{1j?} \frac{\sum_{k'=1}^{K} \pi_{k'|j} \Lambda_{jk'}' I(s \in \{0, 1j, 2k'\})}{\sum_{k'=1}^{K} \pi_{k'|j} \Lambda_{jk'}} - n_{0j?} \frac{\sum_{k'=1}^{K} \pi_{k'|j} \Lambda_{jk'}' I(s \in \{0, 1j, 2k'\})}{1 - \sum_{k'=1}^{K} \pi_{k'|j} \Lambda_{jk'}} \right]$$

and

$$\frac{1}{n} \frac{\partial}{\partial \pi_{k|j}} \ell_{ML}^n(\beta, \pi) = \frac{1}{n} \left[\frac{n_{.jk}}{\pi_{k|j}} - \frac{n_{.j1}}{\pi_{1|j}} + (\Lambda_{jk} - \Lambda_{j1}) \left(\frac{n_{1j?}}{\mu_{j?}} - \frac{n_{0j?}}{1 - \mu_{j?}} \right) \right].$$

For the components of the information matrix we have the general expression

$$I_{\theta_s \theta_t}^{ML}(\beta, \pi, \tau, q) = E_\tau \left(-E_{\beta, \pi, q} \left[\frac{\partial^2}{\partial \theta_s \partial \theta_t} \ell^{ML}(\beta, \pi; Y, X_1, Z_2) \Big| X_1 \right] \right)$$

$$= \sum_{j=1}^{J} - \left(\sum_{k=1}^{K+1} \sum_{y=0}^{1} \frac{\partial^2}{\partial \theta_s \partial \theta_t} \ell^{ML}(\beta, \pi; y, j, k) P_{\beta, \pi, q}(Y = y, Z_2 = k | X_1 = j) \right) \tau_j$$

$$= \sum_{j=1}^{J} - \left[\sum_{k=1}^{K} \left(\frac{\partial^2}{\partial \theta_s \partial \theta_t} \ell^{ML}(\beta, \pi; 1, j, k) q_{1j} \mu_{jk} + \frac{\partial^2}{\partial \theta_s \partial \theta_t} \ell^{ML}(\beta, \pi; 0, j, k) q_{0j}(1 - \mu_{jk}) \right) \pi_{k|j} \right.$$

$$\left. + \frac{\partial^2}{\partial \theta_s \partial \theta_t} \ell^{ML}(\beta, \pi; 1, j, ?)(1 - q_{1j}) \mu_{j?} + \frac{\partial^2}{\partial \theta_s \partial \theta_t} \ell^{ML}(\beta, \pi; 0, j, ?)(1 - q_{0j})(1 - \mu_{j?}) \right] \tau_j.$$

Now we have for $k \neq ?$

$$\frac{\partial^2}{\partial \beta_s \partial \beta_t} \ell^{ML}(\beta, \pi; 1, j, k) q_{1j} \mu_{jk} + \frac{\partial^2}{\partial \beta_s \partial \beta_t} \ell^{ML}(\beta, \pi; 0, j, k) q_{0j}(1 - \mu_{jk})$$

$$= \frac{\mu_{jk}^{st}\mu_{jk} - \mu_{jk}^{s}\mu_{jk}^{t}}{(\mu_{jk})^2}q_{1j}\mu_{jk} - \frac{\mu_{jk}^{st}(1 - \mu_{jk}) + \mu_{jk}^{s}\mu_{jk}^{t}}{(1 - \mu_{jk})^2}q_{0j}(1 - \mu_{jk})$$

$$= \mu_{jk}^{st}(q_{1j} - q_{0j}) - \mu_{jk}^{s}\mu_{jk}^{t}\left(\frac{q_{1j}}{\mu_{jk}} + \frac{q_{0j}}{1 - \mu_{jk}}\right)$$

$$= \mu_{jk}^{st}(q_{1j} - q_{0j}) - \frac{\mu_{jk}^{s}\mu_{jk}^{t}}{\mu_{jk}(1 - \mu_{jk})}[q_{1j}(1 - \mu_{jk}) + q_{0j}\mu_{jk}]$$

and for $k = ?$

$$\frac{\partial^2}{\partial\beta_s\partial\beta_t}\ell^{ML}(\beta, \pi; 1, j, ?)(1 - q_{1j})\mu_{j?} + \frac{\partial^2}{\partial\beta_s\partial\beta_t}\ell^{ML}(\beta, \pi; 0, j, ?)(1 - q_{0j})(1 - \mu_{j?})$$

$$= \mu_{j?}^{st}(q_{0j} - q_{1j}) - \frac{\mu_{j?}^{s}\mu_{j?}^{t}}{\mu_{j?}(1 - \mu_{j?})}[(1 - q_{1j})(1 - \mu_{j?}) + (1 - q_{0j})\mu_{j?}] .$$

Hence we have

$$I_{\beta_s\beta_t}^{ML}(\beta, \pi, \tau, q)$$

$$= \sum_{j=1}^{J}\left[\sum_{k=1}^{K}\left(\frac{\mu_{jk}^{s}\mu_{jk}^{t}}{\mu_{jk}(1 - \mu_{jk})}[q_{1j}(1 - \mu_{jk}) + q_{0j}\mu_{jk}] - \mu_{jk}^{st}(q_{1j} - q_{0j})\right)\pi_{k|j}\right.$$

$$\left. + \frac{\mu_{j?}^{s}\mu_{j?}^{t}}{\mu_{j?}(1 - \mu_{j?})}[(1 - q_{1j})(1 - \mu_{j?}) + (1 - q_{0j})\mu_{j?}] - \mu_{j?}^{st}(q_{0j} - q_{1j})\right]\tau_j .$$

Analogously we have for $k \neq ?$

$$\frac{\partial^2}{\partial\pi_{k'|j'}\partial\pi_{k''|j''}}\ell^{ML}(\beta, \pi; 1, j, k)q_{1j}\mu_{jk} + \frac{\partial^2}{\partial\pi_{k'|j'}\partial\pi_{k''|j''}}\ell^{ML}(\beta, \pi; 0, j, k)q_{0j}(1 - \mu_{jk})$$

$$= \begin{cases} (q_{1j}\mu_{jk} + q_{0j}(1 - \mu_{jk}))(-\frac{1}{\pi_{k|j}^2}) & \text{if } j = j' = j'', k = k' = k'' \\ (q_{1j}\mu_{j1} + q_{0j}(1 - \mu_{j1}))(-\frac{1}{\pi_{1|j}^2}) & \text{if } j = j' = j'', k = 1 \\ 0 & \text{otherwise} \end{cases}$$

and

$$\frac{\partial^2}{\partial\pi_{k'|j'}\partial\pi_{k''|j''}}\ell^{ML}(\beta, \pi; 1, j, ?)(1 - q_{1j})\mu_{j?} + \frac{\partial^2}{\partial\pi_{k'|j'}\partial\pi_{k''|j''}}\ell^{ML}(\beta, \pi; 0, j, ?)(1 - q_{0j})(1 - \mu_{j?})$$

$$= -(\mu_{jk'} - \mu_{j1})(\mu_{jk''} - \mu_{j1})\left(\frac{1 - q_{1j}}{\mu_{j?}} + \frac{1 - q_{0j}}{1 - \mu_{j?}}\right)$$

$$= -(\mu_{jk'} - \mu_{j1})(\mu_{jk''} - \mu_{j1})\frac{(1 - q_{1j})(1 - \mu_{j?}) + (1 - q_{0j})\mu_{j?}}{\mu_{j?}(1 - \mu_{j?})} ;$$

hence for $j' = j'' =: j$

$$I^{ML}_{\pi_{k'|j}, \pi_{k''|j''}}(\beta, \pi, \tau, q)$$

$$= \tau_j \left[\frac{1}{\pi_{1|j}} [q_{1j}\mu_{j1} + q_{0j}(1 - \mu_{j1})] + \frac{1}{\pi_{k'|j}} [q_{1j}\mu_{jk'} + q_{0j}(1 - \mu_{jk'})] I(k' = k'') \right.$$

$$\left. + (\mu_{jk'} - \mu_{j1})(\mu_{jk''} - \mu_{j1}) \frac{(1 - q_{1j})(1 - \mu_{j?}) + (1 - q_{0j})\mu_{j?}}{\mu_{j?}(1 - \mu_{j?})} \right]$$

and $I^{ML}_{\pi_{k'|j}, \pi_{k''|j''}}(\beta, \pi, \tau, q) = 0$ otherwise.
Finally only the terms

$$\frac{\partial^2}{\partial \beta_s \partial \pi_{k|j}} \ell^{ML}(\beta, \pi; 1, j, ?)(1 - q_{1j})\mu_{j?} + \frac{\partial^2}{\partial \beta_s \partial \pi_{k|j}} \ell^{ML}(\beta, \pi; 0, j, ?)(1 - q_{0j})(1 - \mu_{j?})$$

$$= (\mu^s_{jk} - \mu^s_{j1})(q_{0j} - q_{1j}) - \frac{(\mu_{jk} - \mu_{j1})\mu^s_{j?}}{\mu_{j?}(1 - \mu_{j?})}[(1 - q_{1j})(1 - \mu_{j?}) + (1 - q_{0j})\mu_{j?}]$$

contribute to the mixed derivates and hence

$$I^{ML}_{\beta_s \pi_{k|j}}(\beta, \pi, \tau, q)$$

$$= \left[\frac{(\mu_{jk} - \mu_{j1})\mu^s_{j?}}{\mu_{j?}(1 - \mu_{j?})}[(1 - q_{1j})(1 - \mu_{j?}) + (1 - q_{0j})\mu_{j?}] - (\mu^s_{jk} - \mu^s_{j1})(q_{0j} - q_{1j}) \right] \tau_j \; .$$

The formulas simplify if $q_{0j} = q_{1j} =: q_j$. Then we have

$$I^{ML}_{\beta_s \beta_t}(\beta, \pi, \tau, q) = \sum_{j=1}^{J} \left[\left(\sum_{k=1}^{K} \pi_{k|j} \frac{\mu^s_{jk}\mu^t_{jk}}{\mu_{jk}(1 - \mu_{jk})} \right) q_j + \frac{\mu^s_{j?}\mu^t_{j?}}{\mu_{j?}(1 - \mu_{j?})}(1 - q_j) \right] \tau_j$$

$$I^{ML}_{\beta_s \pi_{k|j}}(\beta, \pi, \tau, q) = \tau_j \frac{(\mu_{jk} - \mu_{j1})\mu^s_{j?}}{\mu_{j?}(1 - \mu_{j?})}(1 - q_j)$$

and

$$I^{ML}_{\pi_{k'|j}, \pi_{k''|j''}}(\beta, \pi, \tau, q) = \tau_j \left[\frac{q_j}{\pi_{1|j}} + \frac{q_j}{\pi_{k'|j}} I(k' = k'') + \frac{(\mu_{jk'} - \mu_{j1})(\mu_{jk''} - \mu_{j1})}{\mu_{j?}(1 - \mu_{j?})}(1 - q_j) \right]$$

if $j' = j'' =: j$ and $I^{ML}_{\pi_{k'|j'}, \pi_{k''|j''}}(\beta, \pi, \tau, q) = 0$ otherwise.

Using the approach of Louis (1982) it remains to give a representation for $H_{\theta\theta}(y, j, ?)$. For the single components we have

$$H_{\theta_s \theta_t}(y, j, ?) = Cov \left[\frac{\partial}{\partial \theta_s} \ell^*(\theta; y, j, X_2), \frac{\partial}{\partial \theta_t} \ell^*(\theta; y, j, X_2) \middle| Y = y, X_1 = j, Z_2 = ? \right]$$

$$= \sum_{k=1}^{K} r_{y|j,k}(\theta) \frac{\partial}{\partial \theta_s} \ell^*(\theta; y, j, k) \frac{\partial}{\partial \theta_t} \ell^*(\theta; y, j, k)$$

$$- \left(\sum_{k=1}^{K} r_{y|jk}(\theta) \frac{\partial}{\partial \theta_s} \ell^*(\theta; y, j, k) \right) \left(\sum_{k=1}^{K} r_{y|jk}(\theta) \frac{\partial}{\partial \theta_t} \ell^*(\theta; y, j, k) \right) \; .$$

Appendix B.3

Explicit Representation of the Quantities Used for the Asymptotic Variance of the PML Estimates

The components of $\Sigma_{\widehat{\pi}^n}(\xi)$ are

$$
(\Sigma_{\widehat{\pi}}^n)_{\pi_{k'|j'},\pi_{k''|j''}}(\pi,\tau,q) =
\begin{cases}
0 & \text{if } j \neq j' \\[4pt]
-\dfrac{\pi_{k'|j}\pi_{k''|j}}{\tau_j q_j} & \text{if } j := j' = j'',\, k' \neq k'' \\[6pt]
\dfrac{\pi_{k|j}(1-\pi_{k|j})}{\tau_j q_j} & \text{if } j := j' = j'',\, k := k' = k''
\end{cases}
$$

where we have used the MDX assumption.
For the components of the matrix $J_{\beta p}(\xi^0)$ we have with $\tilde{\pi}^n = \pi(p)$

$$
J_{\beta_s, p_{ijk}}(\beta^0, p^0)
$$

$$
= \frac{\partial}{\partial p_{ijk}} \sum_{j'=1}^{J} \sum_{k'=1}^{K+1} \; p_{1j'k'} \left[\frac{\partial}{\partial \beta_s} \log \mu_{j'k'}(\beta, \pi(p)) \Big|_{\beta^0} \right]
$$

$$
+ p_{0j'k'} \left[\frac{\partial}{\partial \beta_s} \log[1 - \mu_{j'k'}(\beta, \pi(p))] \Big|_{\beta^0} \right] \Big|_{p^0}
$$

$$
= \left[\sum_{j'=1}^{J} \sum_{k'=1}^{K+1} \; p_{1j'k'}^0 \left(\frac{\partial}{\partial p_{ijk}} \frac{\partial}{\partial \beta_s} \log \mu_{j'k'}(\beta, \pi(p)) \Big|_{\beta^0, p^0} \right) \right.
$$

$$
\left. + p_{0j'k'}^0 \left(\frac{\partial}{\partial p_{ijk}} \frac{\partial}{\partial \beta_s} \log[1 - \mu_{j'k'}(\beta, \pi(p))] \Big|_{\beta^0, p^0} \right) \right]
$$

$$
+ \frac{\partial}{\partial \beta_s} \log[\mu_{jk}(\beta)^i (1 - \mu_{jk}(\beta))^{1-i}] \Big|_{\beta^0} \; .
$$

We have $\frac{\partial}{\partial p_{ijk}} \log \mu_{j'k'}(\beta, \pi(p)) \neq 0$ only if $k' =?$ and $j' = j$, hence

$$
\sum_{j'=1}^{J} \sum_{k'=1}^{K+1} \; p_{1j'k'}^0 \left(\frac{\partial}{\partial p_{ijk}} \frac{\partial}{\partial \beta_s} \log \mu_{j'k'}(\beta, \pi(p)) \Big|_{\beta^0, p^0} \right)
$$

$$
+ p_{0j'k'}^0 \left(\frac{\partial}{\partial p_{ijk}} \frac{\partial}{\partial \beta_s} \log[1 - \mu_{j'k'}(\beta, \pi(p))] \Big|_{\beta^0, p^0} \right)
$$

$$
= p_{1j?}^0 \frac{\partial}{\partial p_{ijk}} \frac{\mu_{j?}^s(\beta^0, \pi(p))}{\mu_{j?}(\beta^0, \pi(p))} \Big|_{p^0} - p_{0j?}^0 \frac{\partial}{\partial p_{ijk}} \frac{\mu_{j?}^s(\beta^0, \pi(p))}{1 - \mu_{j?}(\beta^0, \pi(p))} \Big|_{p^0}
$$

$$
= p_{1j?}^0 \frac{[\frac{\partial}{\partial p_{ijk}}\mu_{j?}^s(\beta^0, \pi(p))|_{p^0}]\mu_{j?}(\beta^0, \pi^0) - \mu_{j?}^s(\beta^0, \pi^0)[\frac{\partial}{\partial p_{ijk}}\mu_{j?}(\beta^0, \pi(p))|_{p^0}]}{(\mu_{j?}(\beta^0, \pi^0))^2}
$$

$$
- p_{0j?}^0 \frac{[\frac{\partial}{\partial p_{ijk}}\mu_{j?}^s(\beta^0, \pi(p))|_{p^0}](1 - \mu_{j?}(\beta^0, \pi^0)) + \mu_{j?}^s(\beta^0, \pi^0)[\frac{\partial}{\partial p_{ijk}}\mu_{j?}(\beta^0, \pi(p))|_{p^0}]}{(1 - \mu_{j?}(\beta^0, \pi^0))^2}
$$

$$= p^0_{.j.} \left[\frac{\partial}{\partial p_{ijk}} \mu^s_{j?}(\beta^0, \pi^0) \Big|_{p^0} (q^0_{0j} - q^0_{1j}) \right.$$

$$\left. - \mu^s_{j?}(\beta^0, \pi^0)[\frac{\partial}{\partial p_{ijk}} \mu_{j?}(\beta^0, \pi(p)) \Big|_{p^0}] (\frac{1 - q_{1j}}{\mu_{j?}(\beta^0, \pi^0)} + \frac{1 - q_{0j}}{1 - \mu_{j?}(\beta^0, \pi^0)}) \right]$$

where we have used $p^0_{1j?} = (1 - q_{1j})\mu_{j?}(\beta^0, \pi^0)p^0_{.j.}$ and $p^0_{0j?} = (1 - q_{0j})(1 - \mu_{j?}(\beta^0, \pi^0))p^0_{.j.}$.
Next we have

$$\frac{\partial}{\partial p_{ijk}} \mu_{j?}(\beta^0, \pi(p)) \Big|_{p^0} = \sum_{k'=1}^{K} \Lambda(\beta^0_0 + \beta^0_{1j} + \beta^0_{2k'}) \frac{\partial}{\partial p_{ijk}} \pi_{k'|j}(p) \Big|_{p^0}$$

and

$$\frac{\partial}{\partial p_{ijk}} \mu^s_{j?}(\beta^0, \pi(p)) \Big|_{p^0} = \sum_{k'=1}^{K} \Lambda'(\beta^0_0 + \beta^0_{1j} + \beta^0_{2k'}) I(s \in \{0, 1j, 2k'\}) \frac{\partial}{\partial p_{ijk}} \pi_{k'|j}(p) \Big|_{p^0} .$$

Now

$$\frac{\partial}{\partial p_{ijk}} \pi_{k'|j}(p) \Big|_{p^0} = \frac{\partial}{\partial p_{ijk}} \frac{p_{0j.}\frac{p_{0jk'}}{p_{0j+}} + p_{1j.}\frac{p_{1jk'}}{p_{1j+}}}{p_{.j.}} \Big|_{p^0} = \frac{\frac{\partial}{\partial p_{ijk}} p_{ij.} \frac{p_{ijk'}}{p_{ij+}} \Big|_{p^0} p^0_{.j.} - p^0_{.j.} \pi^0_{k'|j}}{(p^0_{.j.})^2}$$

and

$$\frac{\partial}{\partial p_{ijk}} p_{ij.} \frac{p_{ijk'}}{p_{ij+}} \Big|_{p^0} = \frac{p^0_{ijk'}}{p^0_{ij+}} + p^0_{ij.} \frac{\partial}{\partial p_{ijk}} \frac{p_{ijk'}}{p_{ij+}} \Big|_{p^0}$$

and

$$\frac{\partial}{\partial p_{ijk}} \frac{p_{ijk'}}{p_{ij+}} \Big|_{p^0} = \begin{cases} 0 & \text{if } k = ? \\ \frac{p^0_{ij+} - p^0_{ijk'}}{(p^0_{ij+})^2} & \text{if } k = k' \\ -\frac{p^0_{ijk'}}{(p^0_{ij+})^2} & \text{otherwise} \end{cases} ;$$

hence

$$\frac{\partial}{\partial p_{ijk}} \pi_{k'|j}(p) \Big|_{p^0} = \frac{1}{p^0_{.j.}} \left[\frac{p^0_{ijk'}}{p^0_{ij+}} - \pi^0_{k'|j} + \frac{p^0_{ij.}}{p^0_{ij+}}[I(k = k') - \frac{p^0_{ijk'}}{p^0_{ij+}}]I(k \neq ?) \right].$$

Finally

$$J_{\beta_s, p_{ijk}}(\xi^0)$$

$$= \left\{ \left[\sum_{k'=1}^{K} \Lambda'(\beta_0^0 + \beta_{1j}^0 + \beta_{2k'}^0) I(s \in \{0, 1j, 2k'\}) \right.\right.$$

$$\left(\frac{p_{ijk'}^0}{p_{ij+}^0} - \pi_{k'|j}^0 + \frac{1}{q_{ij}^0}[I(k = k') - \frac{p_{ijk'}^0}{p_{ij+}^0}]I(k \neq ?)) \right] (q_{0j}^0 - q_{1j}^0)$$

$$- \left[\sum_{k'=1}^{K} \Lambda(\beta_0^0 + \beta_{1j}^0 + \beta_{2k'}^0) \left(\frac{p_{ijk'}^0}{p_{ij+}^0} \pi_{k'|j}^0 + \frac{1}{q_{ij}^0}[I(k = k') - \frac{p_{ijk'}^0}{p_{ij+}^0}]I(k \neq ?) \right) \right]$$

$$\mu_{j?}^s(\beta^0, \pi^0) \left(\frac{1 - q_{1j}}{\mu_{j?}(\beta^0, \pi^0)} - \frac{1 - q_{0j}}{1 - \mu_{j?}(\beta^0, \pi^0)} \right) \right\}$$

$$+ \begin{cases} \frac{\mu_{jk}^s(\beta^0, \pi^0)}{\mu_{jk}(\beta^0, \pi^0)} & \text{if } i = 1 \\ -\frac{\mu_{jk}^s(\beta^0, \pi^0)}{1 - \mu_{jk}(\beta^0, \pi^0)} & \text{if } i = 0 \end{cases} .$$

Note that π^0 and q^0 are functions of p^0, which is a function of ξ^0 given by (4.1). The entries of the covariance matrix $\Sigma_p(\xi^0)$ are

$$\left(\Sigma_p(\xi^0) \right)_{p_{ijk} p_{i'j'k'}} = \begin{cases} p_{ijk}^0(1 - p_{ijk}^0) & \text{if } i = i', j = j', k = k' \\ -p_{i'j'k'}^0 p_{ijk}^0 & \text{otherwise} \end{cases} .$$

Appendix B.4

Explicit Representation of the Quantities Used for the Asymptotic Variance of the Estimates Based on the Filling Method

The main task is to yield an explicit representation for the asymptotic variance $\Sigma_{\hat{p}^{*\gamma,n}}$ of the estimate $\hat{p}^{*\gamma,n}$ given by

$$\hat{p}_{ijk}^{*\gamma,n} := n_{ijk} + n_{ij?} \frac{\gamma_{ijk} n_{ijk}}{\sum_{l=1}^{K} \gamma_{ijl} n_{ijl}},$$

used in Section 8. With $\gamma_{ijk} \equiv 1$ we arrive at the estimate used in Section 4.3. In the following we use the abbreviation $as\,Var(d^n)$ for the asymptotic variance of $\sqrt{n}(d^n - d^0)$, where d^n is a consistent estimate for d^0. Similarly we use the abbreviation $asCov(c^n, d^n)$.
Using the expression

$$\hat{p}_{ijk}^{*\gamma,n} = \hat{p}_{ijk}^n (1 + \gamma_{ijk} h_{ij}^{\gamma}(\hat{p}^n)) \quad \text{with } h_{ij}^{\gamma}(p) = \frac{p_{ij?}}{\sum_{l=1}^{K} \gamma_{ijl} p_{ijl}}$$

the delta method yields

$$\begin{aligned}
as\,Var(\hat{p}_{ijk}^{*\gamma,n}) = \quad & (p_{ijk}^0)^2 \, \gamma_{ijk}^2 \; as\,Var(h_{ij}^{\gamma}(\hat{p}^n)) \\
& + [1 + \gamma_{ijk} h_{ij}^{\gamma}(p^0)]^2 \; as\,Var(\hat{p}_{ijk}^n) \\
& + 2 \, p_{ijk}^0 \, [1 + \gamma_{ijk} h_{ij}^{\gamma}(p^0)] \, \gamma_{ijk} \; asCov(\hat{p}_{ijk}^n, h_{ij}^{\gamma}(\hat{p}^n))
\end{aligned}$$

and

$$\begin{aligned}
asCov(\hat{p}_{ijk}^{*\gamma,n}, \hat{p}_{i'j'k'}^{*\gamma,n}) = \quad & p_{ijk}^0 \, \gamma_{ijk} \; asCov(h_{ij}^{\gamma}(\hat{p}^n), h_{i'j'}^{\gamma}(\hat{p}^n)) \, \gamma_{i'j'k'} \, p_{i'j'k'}^0 \\
& + p_{ijk}^0 \, \gamma_{ijk} \; asCov(h_{ij}^{\gamma}(\hat{p}^n), \hat{p}_{i'j'k'}^n) \, [1 + \gamma_{i'j'k'} h_{i'j'}^{\gamma}(p^0)] \\
& + [1 + \gamma_{ijk} h_{ij}^{\gamma}(p^0)] \; asCov(\hat{p}_{ijk}^n, h_{i'j'}^{\gamma}(\hat{p}^n)) \, p_{i'j'k'}^0 \, \gamma_{i'j'k'} \\
& + [1 + \gamma_{ijk} h_{ij}^{\gamma}(p^0)] \; asCov(\hat{p}_{ijk}^n, \hat{p}_{i'j'k'}^n) \, [1 + \gamma_{i'j'k'} h_{i'j'}^{\gamma}(p^0)] .
\end{aligned}$$

Now

$$\frac{\partial}{\partial p_{i'j'k'}} h_{ij}^{\gamma}(p) \Big|_p = \begin{cases} -\dfrac{p_{ij?}}{(\sum_{l=1}^{K} \gamma_{ijl} p_{ijl})^2} \gamma_{i'j'k'} & \text{if } i = i', j = j', k' \neq? \\[3ex] \dfrac{1}{\sum_{l=1}^{K} \gamma_{ijl} p_{ijl}} & \text{if } i = i', j = j', k' =? \\[3ex] 0 & \text{otherwise} \end{cases}$$

hence the delta method yields

$$as\,Var(h_{ij}^\gamma(\widehat{p}^n)) = \sum_{k=1}^{K+1}\sum_{k'=1}^{K+1} \frac{\partial}{\partial p_{ijk}}h_{ij}^\gamma(p)\Big|_{p^0}\, asCov(\widehat{p}_{ijk}^n, \widehat{p}_{ijk'}^n)\, \frac{\partial}{\partial p_{ijk'}}h_{ij}^\gamma(p)\Big|_{p^0}$$

$$= \sum_{k=1}^{K+1} \frac{\partial}{\partial p_{ijk}}h_{ij}^\gamma(p)\Big|_{p^0}\, p_{ijk}^0\, \frac{\partial}{\partial p_{ijk}}h_{ij}^\gamma(p)\Big|_{p^0} - \sum_{k=1}^{K+1}\sum_{k'=1}^{K+1} \frac{\partial}{\partial p_{ijk}}h_{ij}^\gamma(p)\Big|_{p^0}\, p_{ijk}^0 p_{ijk'}^0\, \frac{\partial}{\partial p_{ijk'}}h_{ij}^\gamma(p)\Big|_{p^0}$$

$$= \frac{1}{(\sum_{l=1}^{K}\gamma_{ijl}p_{ijl}^0)^2}\left[\frac{(p_{ij?}^0)^2}{(\sum_{l=1}^{K}\gamma_{ijl}p_{ijl}^0)^2}\left(\sum_{k=1}^{K}\gamma_{ijk}^2 p_{ijk}^0\right) + p_{ij?}^0\right.$$

$$- \frac{(p_{ij?}^0)^2}{(\sum_{l=1}^{K}\gamma_{ijl}p_{ijl}^0)^2}\left(\sum_{k=1}^{K}\sum_{k'=1}^{K}\gamma_{ijk}p_{ijk}^0 p_{ijk'}^0\gamma_{ijk'}\right)$$

$$+ 2\frac{p_{ij?}^0}{\sum_{l=1}^{K}\gamma_{ijl}p_{ijl}^0}\left(\sum_{k=1}^{K} p_{ijk}^0 p_{ij?}^0\gamma_{ijk}\right) - (p_{ij?}^0)^2\right]$$

$$= \frac{1}{(\sum_{l=1}^{K}\gamma_{ijl}p_{ijl}^0)^2}\left[\left(\frac{p_{ij?}^0}{\sum_{l=1}^{K}\gamma_{ijl}p_{ijl}^0}\right)^2\left(\sum_{k=1}^{K}\gamma_{ijk}^2 p_{ijk}^0\right) + p_{ij?}^0\right]$$

and for $i \neq i'$ or $j \neq j'$ we have

$$asCov(h_{ij}^\gamma(\widehat{p}^n), h_{i'j'}^\gamma(\widehat{p}^n)) = 0$$

Further we have

$$asCov(\widehat{p}_{ijk}^n, h_{i'j'}^\gamma(\widehat{p}^n)) = \sum_{l=1}^{K+1} asCov(\widehat{p}_{ijk}^n, \widehat{p}_{i'j'l}^n)\frac{\partial}{\partial p_{i'j'l}}h_{i'j'}^\gamma(p)\Big|_{p^0}$$

hence for $i \neq i'$ and $j \neq j'$

$$asCov(\widehat{p}_{ijk}^n, h_{i'j'}^\gamma(\widehat{p}^n))$$

$$= -\frac{1}{\sum_{l=1}^{K}\gamma_{i'j'l}p_{i'j'l}^0}\left[\left(\sum_{l=1}^{K} p_{ijk}^0 p_{i'j'l}^0\frac{p_{i'j'?}^0}{\sum_{l=1}^{K}\gamma_{i'j'l}p_{i'j'l}^0}\gamma_{i'j'l}\right) - p_{ijk}^0 p_{i'j'?}^0\right] = 0$$

and

$$asCov(\widehat{p}_{ijk}^n, h_{ij}^\gamma(\widehat{p}^n)) = \frac{1}{\sum_{l=1}^{K}\gamma_{ijl}p_{ijl}^0}\left[-p_{ijk}^0\frac{p_{ij?}^0}{\sum_{l=1}^{K}\gamma_{ijl}p_{ijl}^0}\gamma_{ijk}\right] = -\frac{\gamma_{ijk}}{\sum_{l=1}^{K}\gamma_{ijl}p_{ijl}^0}p_{ijk}^0 h_{ij}^\gamma(p^0)$$

So we have

$$as\,Var(\widehat{p}_{ijk}^{*\gamma,n}) = (p_{ijk}^0)^2\frac{\gamma_{ijk}^2}{(\sum_{l=1}^{K}\gamma_{ijl}p_{ijl}^0)^2}\left[(h_{ij}^\gamma(p^0))^2\left(\sum_{l=1}^{K}\gamma_{ijl}^2 p_{ijl}^0\right) + p_{ij?}^0\right]$$

$$+ [1 + \gamma_{ijk} h_{ij}^\gamma(p^0)]^2 p_{ijk}^0 (1 - p_{ijk}^0)$$

$$- 2(p_{ijk}^0)^2 \gamma_{ijk}^2 [1 + \gamma_{ijk} h_{ij}^\gamma(p^0)] \frac{h_{ij}^\gamma(p^0)}{\sum_{l=1}^K \gamma_{ijl} p_{ijl}^0}$$

and

$$asCov(\hat{\tilde{p}}_{ijk}^{*\gamma,n}, \hat{\tilde{p}}_{ijk'}^{*\gamma,n}) = p_{ijk}^0 \gamma_{ijk} \frac{1}{(\sum_{l=1}^K \gamma_{ijl} p_{ijl}^0)^2} \left[(h_{ij}^\gamma(p^0))^2 \left(\sum_{l=1}^K \gamma_{ijl}^2 p_{ijl}^0 \right) + p_{ij?}^0 \right] \gamma_{ijk'} p_{ijk'}^0$$

$$- p_{ijk}^0 \gamma_{ijk} \frac{\gamma_{ijk'}}{\sum_{l=1}^K \gamma_{ijl} p_{ijl}^0} p_{ijk'}^0 h_{ij}^\gamma(p^0)[1 + \gamma_{ijk'} h_{ij}^\gamma(p^0)]$$

$$- [1 + \gamma_{ijk} h_{ij}^\gamma(p^0)] \frac{\gamma_{ijk}}{\sum_{l=1}^K \gamma_{ijl} p_{ijl}^0} p_{ijk}^0 h_{ij}^\gamma(p^0) p_{ijk'}^0 \gamma_{ijk'}$$

$$- [1 + \gamma_{ijk} h_{ij}^\gamma(p^0)] p_{ijk}^0 p_{ijk'}^0 [1 + \gamma_{ijk'} h_{ij}^\gamma(p^0)]$$

$$= p_{ijk}^0 p_{ijk'}^0 \gamma_{ijk} \gamma_{ijk'}$$

$$\left\{ \frac{1}{(\sum_{l=1}^K \gamma_{ijl} p_{ijl}^0)^2} \left[(h_{ij}^\gamma(p^0))^2 \left(\sum_{l=1}^K \gamma_{ijl}^2 p_{ijl}^0 \right) + p_{ij?}^0 \right] \right.$$

$$\left. - 2 \frac{h_{ij}^\gamma(p^0)}{\sum_{l=1}^K \gamma_{ijl} p_{ijl}^0} - (\gamma_{ijk} + \gamma_{ijk'}) \frac{(h_{ij}^\gamma(p^0))^2}{\sum_{l=1}^K \gamma_{ijl} p_{ijl}^0} \right\}$$

$$- p_{ijk}^{*0} p_{ijk'}^{*0}$$

and for $i \neq i'$ and $j \neq j'$ we have

$$asCov(\hat{\tilde{p}}_{ijk}^{*\gamma,n}, \hat{\tilde{p}}_{i'j'k'}^{*\gamma,n}) = -[1 + \gamma_{ijk} h_{ij}^\gamma(p^0)] p_{ijk}^0 p_{i'j'k'}^0 [1 + \gamma_{i'j'k'} h_{i'j'}^\gamma(p^0)]$$

$$= p_{ijk}^{*0} p_{i'j'k'}^{*0} .$$

If we use the Filling method under the MAR assumption, i.e., if $\gamma_{ijk} \equiv 1$, then we arrive at

$$asVar(\hat{\tilde{p}}_{ijk}^{*n}) = (p_{ijk}^0)^2 \frac{1}{(p_{ij+}^0)^2} \left[\left(\frac{p_{ij?}^0}{p_{ij+}^0} \right)^2 p_{ij+}^0 + p_{ij?}^0 \right]$$

$$+ \left(1 + \frac{p_{ij?}^0}{p_{ij+}^0} \right)^2 p_{ijk}^0 (1 - p_{ijk}^0) - 2(p_{ijk}^0)^2 \left(1 + \frac{p_{ij?}^0}{p_{ij+}^0} \right) \frac{p_{ij?}^0}{(p_{ij+}^0)^2}$$

$$= p_{ijk}^{*0} \left[\frac{p_{ij?}^0}{(p_{ij+}^0)^2} p_{ijk}^0 + \left(1 + \frac{p_{ij?}^0}{p_{ij+}^0} \right) (1 - p_{ijk}^0) - 2 p_{ijk}^0 \frac{p_{ij?}^0}{(p_{ij+}^0)^2} \right]$$

$$= p_{ijk}^{*0} \left[1 + \frac{p_{ij?}^0}{p_{ij+}^0} - p_{ijk}^{*0} - p_{ijk}^0 \frac{p_{ij?}^0}{(p_{ij+}^0)^2} \right]$$

$$= p_{ijk}^{*0}(1 - p_{ijk}^{*0}) + p_{ijk}^0 \left(1 + \frac{p_{ij?}^0}{p_{ij+}^0} \right) \frac{p_{ij?}^0}{p_{ij+}^0} \left(1 - \frac{p_{ijk}^0}{p_{ij+}^0} \right)$$

$$= p_{ijk}^{*0}(1 - p_{ijk}^{*0}) + \left(1 + \frac{p_{ij?}^0}{p_{ij+}^0} \right) p_{ij?}^0 \frac{p_{ijk}^0}{p_{ij+}^0} \left(1 - \frac{p_{ijk}^0}{p_{ij+}^0} \right)$$

and

$$asCov(\widehat{p}_{ijk}^{*n}, \widehat{p}_{i'k'}^{*n}) = p_{ijk}^0 p_{ijk'}^0 \left\{ \frac{1}{(p_{ij+}^0)^2} \left[\frac{(p_{ij?}^0)^2}{(p_{ij+}^0)^2} p_{ij+}^0 + p_{ij?}^0 \right] - 2\frac{p_{ij?}^0}{(p_{ij+}^0)^2} - 2\frac{(p_{ij?}^0)^2}{(p_{ij+}^0)^3} \right\}$$

$$- p_{ijk}^{*0} p_{ijk'}^{*0}$$

$$= -p_{ijk}^{*0} p_{ijk'}^{*0} + p_{ijk}^0 p_{ijk'}^0 \left[\frac{p_{ij?}^0}{(p_{ij+}^0)^2} \left(1 + \frac{p_{ij?}^0}{p_{ij+}^0} \right) - 2\frac{p_{ij?}^0}{(p_{ij+}^0)^2} \left(1 + \frac{p_{ij?}^0}{p_{ij+}^0} \right) \right]$$

$$= -p_{ijk}^{*0} p_{ijk'}^{*0} - p_{ijk}^0 p_{ijk'}^0 \frac{p_{ij?}^0}{(p_{ij+}^0)^2} \left(1 + \frac{p_{ij?}^0}{p_{ij+}^0} \right)$$

$$= -p_{ijk}^{*0} p_{ijk'}^{*0} - \left(1 + \frac{p_{ij?}^0}{p_{ij+}^0} \right) p_{ij?}^0 \frac{p_{ijk}^0}{p_{ij+}^0} \frac{p_{ijk'}^0}{p_{ij+}^0}$$

and for $i \neq i'$ and $j \neq j'$

$$asCov(\widehat{p}_{ijk}^{*n}, \widehat{p}_{i'j'k'}^{*n}) = -p_{ijk}^{*0} p_{i'j'k'}^{*0} .$$

It remains to consider the entries of the matrix $H_{\beta p*}(\beta, p^*)$, which are given by

$$H_{\beta_s, p_{ijk}^*}(\beta, p^*) = \frac{\partial}{\partial p_{ijk}^*} \left\{ \sum_{j'=1}^J \sum_{k'=1}^K \left[p_{1j'k'}^*[1 - \Lambda(\beta_0 + \beta_{1j'} + \beta_{2k'})] \right. \right.$$

$$\left. \left. -p_{0j'k'}^* \Lambda(\beta_0 + \beta_{1j'} + \beta_{2k'}) \right] I(s \in \{0, 1j', 2k'\}) \right\}$$

$$= I(s \in \{0, 1j, 2k\}) \begin{cases} -\Lambda(\beta_0 + \beta_{1j} + \beta_{2k}) & \text{if } i = 0 \\ 1 - \Lambda(\beta_0 + \beta_{1j} + \beta_{2k}) & \text{if } i = 1 \end{cases}$$

References

Afifi, A.A. & Elashoff, R.M. (1966) *Missing observations in multivariate statistics I. Review of the literature.* Journal of the American Statistical Association 61, 595-604

Aitkin, M. & Wilson, G.T. (1980) *Mixture models, outliers, and the EM algorithm.* Technometrics 22, 325-331

Baker, S.G., Rosenberger, W.F., & Dersimonian, R. (1992) *Closed-form estimates for missing counts in two-way contingency tables.* Statistics in Medicine 11, 643-657

Bartlett, M.S. (1937) *Some examples of statistical methods of research in agriculture and applied biology.* Journal of the Royal Statistical Society B 4, 137-170

Beale, E.M.L. & Little, R.J.A. (1975) *Missing values in multivariate analysis.* Journal of the Royal Statistical Society B 37, 129-145

Benichou, J. & Gail, M.H. (1989) *A delta method for implicitly defined random variables.* The American Statistician 43, 41-44

Blackhurst, D.W. & Schluchter, M.D. (1989) *Logistic regression with a partially observed covariate.* Communications in Statistics – Simulation and Computation 18, 163-177

Blettner, M. (1987) *Verallgemeinerte Risikofunktionen bei der Auswertung epidemiologischer Studien zur Beurteilung des Krebsrisikos nach Strahlenexposition.* Ph.D. thesis, Department of Statistics, University of Dortmund (in German)

Boice, J.D., Blettner, M., Kleinerman, R., et al. (1989) *Radiation dose and breast cancer risk in patients treated for cancer of the cervix.* International Journal of Cancer 44, 7-14

Breslow, N.E. & Cain, K.C. (1988) *Logistic regression for two-stage case-control data.* Biometrika 75, 11-20

Breslow, N.E. & Day, N.E. (1980) *Statistical methods in cancer research, vol. 1 – The analysis of case-control studies.* IARC Scientific Publications No. 32, Lyon

Buck, S.F. (1960) *A method of estimation of missing values in multivariate data suitable for use with an electronic computer.* Journal of the Royal Statistical Society B 22, 302-306

Byar, D.P. & Gail, M.H. (1989) *Introduction. Errors-in-Variables Workshop.* Statistics in Medicine 8, 1027-1029

Carroll, R.J. (1992) *Approaches to estimation with errors in predictors.* In: *Advances in GLIM and Statistical Modelling,* ed. by Fahrmeier, L., Francis, B., Gilchrist, R., Tutz, G., Lecture Notes in Statistics 78, Springer, 40-47

Carroll, R.J., Spiegelman, C.H., Lan, K.K.G., Bailey, K.T., and Abbott, R.D. (1984) *On errors-in-variables for binary regression models.* Biometrika 71, 19-25

Carroll, R.J. & Wand, M.P. (1991) *Semiparametric estimation in logistic measurement error models.* Journal of the Royal Statistical Society B 53, 573-585

Chow, W.K. (1979) *A look at various estimators in logistic models in the presence of missing values.* Proceedings of the American Statistical Association, Business and Economics Statistics Section, 417-420

Cochran, W.G. (1977) *Sampling Techniques.* 3rd edition, Wiley, New York

Commenges, D., Gagnon M., Letenneur, L., Dartigues, J.F., Barbarger-Gateau, P., & Salamon R. (1992) *Improving screening for dementia in the elderly using mini-mental state examination subcores, Benton's visual retention test, and Isaacs' set test.* Epidemiology 3, 185-188

Cox, D.R. (1972) *Regression models and life tables (with discussion).* Journal of the Royal Statistical Society B 34, 187-220

Dagenais, M.G. (1973) *The use of observations in the multiple regression analysis: A generalized least squares approach.* Journal of Econometrics 1, 317-328

Dempster, A.P., Laird, N.M., & Rubin, D.B. (1977) *Maximum likelihood estimation from incomplete data via EM algorithm (with discussion).* Journal of the Royal Statistical Society

B 39, 1-38

Dodge, Y. (1985) *Analysis of experiments with missing data.* Wiley, New York

Flanders, W.D. & Greenland, S. (1991) *Analytic methods for two-stage case-control studies and other stratified designs.* Statistics in Medicine 10, 739-747

Fuchs, C. (1982) *Maximum likelihood estimation and model selection in contingency tables with missing data.* Journal of the American Statistical Association 77, 270-278

Gail, M.H., Wieand, S., & Piantadosi, S. (1984) *Biased estimation of treatment effect in randomized experiments with nonlinear regressions and omitted covariates.* Biometrika 71, 431-444

Gill, R.D. (1986) *A note on some methods for regression analysis with incomplete observations.* Sankhya B 48, 19-30

Gong, G. & Samaniego, F.J. (1981) *Pseudo maximum likelihood estimation: Theory and application.* Annals of Statistics 9, 861-869

Hansen, M.H. & Hurwitz, W.N. (1946) *The problem of non-response in sample surveys.* Journal of the American Statistical Association 41, 517-529

Heitjan, D.F. (1989) *Inference from grouped continuous data: A review.* Statistical Science 4, 164-183

Hill, R.C. & Ziemer, R.F. (1983) *Missing regressor values under conditions of multicollinearity.* Communications in Statistics – Theory and Methods 12, 2557-2573

Ibrahim, J.G. (1990) *Incomplete data in generalized linear models.* Journal of the American Statistical Association 85, 765-769

Ibrahim, J.G. & Weisberg, S. (1992) *Incomplete data in generalized linear models with continuous covariates.* Australian Journal of Statistics 34, 461-470

Illi, S. (1993) *Fehlende Werte in Kontingenztafeln.* Diploma thesis, Department of Statistics, Ludwig Maximilian University, Munich (in German)

Jarrett, R.G. (1978) *The analysis of designed experiments with missing observations.* Applied Statistics 27, 38-46

Lehmann, E.L. (1983) *Theory of point estimation.* Wiley, New York

Little, R.J.A. (1982) *Models for nonresponse in sample surveys.* Journal of the American Statistical Association 77, 237-250

Little, R.J.A. (1983) *The nonignorable case.* In: *Incomplete data in sample surveys, Vol. 2,* ed. by Madow, W.G., Olkin, I., & Rubin, D.B., Academic Press, New York, 383-413

Little, R.J.A. (1992) *Regression with missing X's: A review.* Journal of the American Statistical Association 87, 1227-1237

Little, R.J.A. & Rubin, D.B. (1987) *Statistical analysis with missing data.* Wiley, New York

Little, R.J.A. & Schluchter, M.D. (1985) *Maximum likelihood estimation for mixed continuous and categorical data with missing values.* Biometrika 72, 497-512

Louis, T.A. (1982) *Finding the observed information matrix when using the EM algorithm.* Journal of the Royal Statistical Society B 44, 226-233

Marshall, J.R. (1989) *The use of dual or multiple reports in epidemiological studies.* Statistics in Medicine 8, 1041-1049

Miettinen, O.S. (1985) *Theoretical epidemiology.* Wiley, New York

Newey, W.K. (1990) *Semiparametric efficiency bounds.* Journal of Applied Econometrics 5, 99-135

Nijman, T. & Palm, F. (1988) *Efficiency gains due to using missing data procedures in regression models.* Statistical Papers 29, 249-256

Nordheim, E.V. (1984) *Inference from nonrandomly missing categorical data: An example from a genetic study on Turner's syndrome.* Journal of the American Statistical Association 79, 772-780

Oh, H.L. & Scheuren, F.J. (1983) *Weighting adjustment for unit nonresponse.* In: *Incomplete data in sample surveys, Vol. 2,* ed. by Madow, W.G., Olkin, I., & Rubin, D.B., Academic Press, New York, 143-184

Parke, W.R. (1986) *Pseudo maximum likelihood estimation: The asymptotic distribution.* Annals of Statistics 14, 355-357

Pepe, M.S. & Fleming, T.R. (1991) *A nonparametric method for dealing with mismeasured covariate data.* Journal of the American Statistical Association 86, 108-113

Pfanzagl, J. (1990) *Estimation in Semiparametric Models.* Lecture Notes in Statistics 63, Springer

Pfisterer, J., Kommoss, F., Renz, H., et al. *Prognostic influence of flow cytometric analysis of nuclear DNA content in advanced ovarian cancer.* unpublished

Philipps, M.J (1993) *Contingency tables with missing data.* The Statistician 42, 9-18

Pierce, D.A. (1982) *The asymptotic effect of substituting estimators for parameters in certain types of statistics.* Annals of Statistics 10, 475-478

Pregibon, D. (1977) *Typical survey data: Estimation and imputation.* Survey Methodology 2, 79-102

Prentice R.L. (1982) *Covariate measurement errors and parametric estimation in the failure time regression model.* Biometrika 69, 331-342

Pugh, M., Robins, J., Lipsitz, S. & Harrington, D. (1993) *Inference in the Cox proportional hazards model with missing covariate data.* Technical report 758Z, Division of Biostatistics, Dana-Farber Cancer Institute, Boston

Randles, R.H. (1982) *On the asymptotic normality of statistics with estimated parameters.* Annals of Statistics 10, 462-474

Rao, P.S.R.S. (1983) *Randomization approach.* In: *Incomplete data in sample surveys, Vol. 2,* ed. by Madow, W.G., Olkin, I., & Rubin, D.B., Academic Press, New York, 97-106

Reilly, M. (1991) *Semi-parametric methods of dealing with missing or surrogate covariate data.* Ph.D. thesis, Dept. of Biostatistics, University of Washington, Seattle

Reilly, M. & Pepe, M. (1993a) *A Mean Score method for missing and auxiliary covariate data in regression models.* Biometrika (submitted)

Reilly, M. & Pepe, M. (1993b) *Inference with incomplete covariates using hot deck multiple imputation.* Journal of the American Statistical Association (submitted)

Robins, J.M. & Rotnitzky, A. (1992) *Recovery of information and adjustment for dependent censoring using surrogate markers.* In: *AIDS epidemiology – Methodological issues,* ed. by Jewell, N.P., Dietz, K., and Farewell, V.T., Birkhäuser, Boston, 297-331

Robinson, L.D. & Jewell, N.P. (1991) *Some surprising results about covariate adjustment in logistic regression models.* International Statistical Review 59, 227-240

Rosenbaum, P.R. (1987) *Model-based direct adjustment.* Journal of the American Statistical Association 82, 387-394

Rubin, D.B. (1976) *Inference and missing data.* Biometrika 63, 581-592

Rubin, D.B. (1987) *Multiple imputation for nonresponse in surveys.* Wiley, New York

Schafer, D.W. (1987) *Covariate measurement error in generalized linear models.* Biometrika 74, 385-391

Schemper, M. & Smith, T.L. (1990) *Efficient evaluation of treatment effects in the presence of missing covariate values.* Statistics in Medicine 9, 777-784

Schick, A. & Susarla, V. (1988) *Efficient estimation in some missing data problems.* Journal of Statistical Planning and Inference 19, 217-228

Schill, W., Jöckel, K.H., Drescher, K., & Timm, J. (1993) *Logistic analysis in case-control studies under validation sampling.* Biometrika 80, 339-352

Stone, C.J. (1977) *Consistent nonparametric regression.* Annals of Statistics 5, 595-645

Storm, H.H., Anderson M., Boice J.D. Blettner, M., Stovall, M., Mouridsen H.T., Domber-nowsky, P., Rose, C., Jacobsen, A. & Pederson M. (1992) *Adjuvant radiotherapy and risk of contralateral breast cancer.* Journal of the National Cancer Institute 84, 1245-1250

Tanner, M.A. (1991) *Tools for statistical inference.* Lecture Notes in Statistics 67, Springer, New York

Thompson, R. & Baker, R.J. (1981) *Composite link functions in generalized linear models.* Applied Statistics 30, 125-131

Toutenburg, H. & Walther, W. (1992) *Statistische Behandlung unvollständiger Datensätze.* Deutsche Zahnärztliche Zeitschrift 47, 104-106 (in German)

Vach, W. (1994) *Missing values: Statistical theory and computational practice.* In: *Computational statistics. Papers collected on the occasion of the 25th conference on statistical computing at Schloß Reisensburg,* ed. by Dirschedl, P. & Ostermann, R., Physika Verlag, to appear

Vach, W. & Blettner, M. (1991) *Biased estimation of the odds ratio in case-control studies due to the use of ad-hoc methods of correcting for missing values for confounding variables.* American Journal of Epidemiology 134, 895-907

Vach, W. & Blettner, M. (1994) *Logistic regression with incompletely observed categorical covariates – Investigating the sensitivity against violation of the missing at random assumption.* Statistics in Medicine (submitted)

Vach, W. & Schumacher, M. (1992) *Logistic regression with incompletely observed categorical covariates.* In: *Data analysis and statistical inference. Festschrift in honour of Friedhelm Eicker,* ed. by Schach, S. & Trenkler, G., Verlag Josef Eul, Bergisch Gladbach, 219-238

Vach, W. & Schumacher, M. (1993) *Logistic regression with incompletely observed categorical covariates – A comparison of three approaches.* Biometrika 80, 353-362

Walker, A.M. & Lanes, S.F. (1991) *Misclassification of covariates.* Statistics in Medicine 10, 1181-1196

Wedderburn, R.W.M. (1974) *Quasi-likelihood functions, generalized linear models, and the Gauss-Newton method.* Biometrika 61, 439-447

White, J.E. (1982) *A two-stage design for the study of the relationship between a rare exposure and a rare disease.* American Journal of Epidemiology 115, 119-128

Whittemore, A.S. & Grosser, S. (1986) *Regression methods for data with incomplete covariates.* In: *Modern statistical methods in chronic disease epidemiology,* ed. by Moolgavkar, S.H. & Prentice, R.L., Wiley-Interscience, New York, 19-34

Wild, C.J. (1991) *Fitting prospective regression models to case-control data.* Biometrika 78, 705-717

Wilks, S.S. (1932) *Moments and distributions of estimates of population parameters from fragmentary samples.* Annals of Mathematical Statistics 3, 163-195

Willett, W. (1989) *An overview of issues related to the correction of non-differential exposure measurement error in epidemiological studies.* Statistics in Medicine 8, 1031-1040

Wu, C.F.J. (1983) *On the convergence properties of the EM algorithm.* Annals of Statistics 11, 95-103

Yates, F. (1933) *The analysis of replicated experiments when the field results are incomplete.* Empire Journal Of Experimental Agriculture 1, 129-142

Yuen Fung, K. & Wrobel, B.A. (1989) *The treatment of missing values in logistic regression.* Biometrical Journal 31, 35-47

Zeger, S.L. & Liang, K.Y. (1992) *An overview of methods for the analysis of longitudinal data.* Statistics in Medicine 11, 1825-1839

Zhao, L.P. & Lipsitz, S. (1992) *Designs and analysis of two-stage designs.* Statistics in Medicine 11, 769-782

Zhou, H. & Pepe, M.S. (1993) *Auxiliary covariate data in failure time regression.* **Biometrika** (submitted)

Notation Index

Subject Index

General Remarks

Lecture Notes are printed by photo-offset from the master-copy delivered in camera-ready form by the authors of monographs, resp. editors of proceedings volumes. For this purpose Springer-Verlag provides technical instructions for the preparation of manuscripts. Volume editors are requested to distribute these to all contributing authors of proceedings volumes. Some homogeneity in the presentation of the contributions in a multi-author volume is desirable.

Careful preparation of manuscripts will help keep production time short and ensure a satisfactory appearance of the finished book. The actual production of a Lecture Notes volume normally takes approximately 8 weeks.

For monograph manuscripts typed or typeset according to our instructions, Springer-Verlag can, if necessary, contribute towards the preparation costs at a fixed rate.

Authors of monographs receive 50 free copies of their book. Editors of proceedings volumes similarly receive 50 copies of the book and are responsible for redistributing these to authors etc. at their discretion. No reprints of individual contributions can be supplied. No royalty is paid on Lecture Notes volumes.

Volume authors and editors are entitled to purchase further copies of their book for their personal use at a discount of 33.3% and other Springer mathematics books at a discount of 20% directly from Springer-Verlag. Authors contributing to proceedings volumes may purchase the volume in which their article appears at a discount of 20 %.

Springer-Verlag secures the copyright for each volume.

Series Editors:

Professor S. Fienberg
Department of Statistics
Carnegie Mellon University
Pittsburgh, Pennsylvania 15213
USA

Professor J. Gani
Department of Statistics IAS
Australian National University
GPO Box 4
Canberra ACT 2601
Australia

Professor K. Krickeberg
3 Rue de L'Estrapade
75005 Paris
France

Professor I. Olkin
Department of Statistics
Stanford University
Stanford, California 94305
USA

Professor N. Wermuth
Department of Psychology
Johannes Gutenberg University
Postfach 3980
D-6500 Mainz
Germany